POCKET

PHYSICAL
DIAGNOSIS

POCKET GUIDE TO

PHYSICAL DIAGNOSIS

JANICE L. WILLMS, M.D., Ph.D.
Institute of Medicine and Humanities
St. Patrick Hospital and The University of Montana
Missoula, Montana

HENRY SCHNEIDERMAN, M.D., F.A.C.P.
Associate Professor of Medicine (Geriatrics) and Pathology
University of Connecticut Health Center
Farmington, Connecticut
Physician-in-Chief
Hebrew Home & Hospital
West Hartford, Connecticut

Illustrations by:
Joyce Lavery

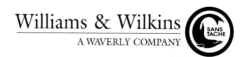

Williams & Wilkins
A WAVERLY COMPANY

BALTIMORE • PHILADELPHIA • LONDON • PARIS • BANGKOK
BUENOS AIRES • HONG KONG • MUNICH • SYDNEY • TOKYO • WROCLAW

Editor: Timothy S. Satterfield
Managing Editor: Crystal Taylor
Production Coordinator: Carol Eckhart
Copy Editor: Bill Cady
Designer: Laura O'Leary
Illustration Planner: Ray Lowman
Typesetter: Cynthia E. Council
Printer & Binder: R.R. Donnelley & Sons

351 West Camden Street
Baltimore, Maryland 21201-2436 USA

Rose Tree Corporate Center
1400 North Providence Road
Building II, Suite 5025
Media, Pennsylvania 19063-2043 USA

Printed in the United States of America

Library of Congress Cataloging-in-Publication Data

Willms, Janice L.
  Pocket guide to physical diagnosis/Janice L. Willms, Henry Schneiderman; illustrations
by Joyce Lavery.
   p. cm.
  Includes bibliographical references and index.
  ISBN 0-683-09116-6
  1. Physical diagnosis—Handbooks, manuals, etc. I. Schneiderman, Henry, 1951–   .
II. Title.
  [DNLM: 1. Physical Examination—handbooks. WB 39 W738p 1996]
RC76.W553 1996
616.07'54—dc20
DNLM/DLC
for Library of Congress
                                          95-33622
                                            CIP

96 97 98 99
1 2 3 4 5 6 7 8 9 10

ISBN 0-683-09116-6

9 780683 091168
90000

Preface

"Why is it that medical textbooks must weigh so much and be so bulky?" asks a weary clinical clerk as she shifts a heavy pack from one shoulder to the other. Why, indeed? Simply because there is so much information requisite to a comprehensive textbook such as *Physical Diagnosis: Bedside Evaluation of Diagnosis and Function,* the classroom counterpart to this pocket-sized guide.

The student of clinical assessment and physical diagnosis must possess and study a detailed textbook, as must the practicing clinician who needs reminder and reinforcement of infrequently used techniques or review of the pathoanatomic and pathophysiologic bases of abnormal physical signs. There are times in clinical clerkships and houseofficerships, however, when nothing serves better than a highly streamlined listing of goals, techniques, and interpretations of those variants of history and examination that, unlike the basic framework, have not been committed to memory. Such an outline in the pocket of the white coat and then in hand allows instant bedside or office consultation; that is how the particular physical diagnosis special maneuver can be performed and interpreted correctly, right then and there, with the patient still present.

This little volume is our contribution to the "external brain" collections that we all carry when we leave our offices for the wards and other places where our patients await. We hope you work *Pocket Guide to Physical Diagnosis* hard, to make maximal and optimal use of the subtle, varied, and uniquely human and humane skills of the clinical encounter. We all learn medicine by doing, by practice, and this applies to seasoned doctors as much as to our younger colleagues. May this book enhance your practice.

JANICE L. WILLMS
HENRY SCHNEIDERMAN

Contents

Preface vii

chapter 1
**TWO TIERS OF INVESTIGATION: THE SCREENING
AND EXTENDED EXAMINATIONS** 1
  Screening or Comprehensive Examination 1
  Extended or Problem-Focused Examination 14

chapter 2
GENERAL APPEARANCE AND VITAL SIGNS 33

chapter 3
EXAMINATION OF THE SKIN 47

chapter 4
**HEAD, EYES, EARS, NOSE, ORAL CAVITY,
AND THROAT** 67

chapter 5
NECK 99

chapter 6
BREASTS AND AXILLAE 115

chapter 7
THORAX AND LUNGS 125

chapter 8
HEART AND GREAT VESSELS 141

chapter 9
ABDOMEN 169

chapter 10
LIMBS 193

chapter 11
NEUROLOGIC EXAMINATION 227

chapter 12
LOWER BACK 251

chapter 13
MALE GENITALIA AND RECTUM 265

chapter 14
FEMALE GENITALIA AND RECTUM 277

Figure and Table Credits 295

Index 297

1

Two Tiers of Investigation: The Screening and Extended Examinations

SCREENING (COMPREHENSIVE) MEDICAL HISTORY

The medical history is the story of illness, disability, or deviation from normality as defined by the patient. Your role as medical interviewer is to guide the teller through the details of health and illness without subverting the "facts" as the patient presents them.

In terms of process, an effective medical interview is facilitated by
- A private, quiet, and comfortable place to meet
- Use of effective verbal and nonverbal behaviors
    - Nonverbal
        - Body language, to include appropriate distance, relative positions, and avoidance of distracting habits
        - Eye contact
        - Positive reinforcement, to include showing interest, encouragement, physical contact when appropriate, and empathic modes
    - Verbal
        - Careful use of open and closed questions
        - Avoidance of jargon
        - Avoidance of unnecessary duplication of questions
        - Effective use of silence
        - Pacing appropriate to the situation

- Ability to be attentive to the patient's agenda without losing control of the medical goals of the interview (Table 1.1)

By convention, the formal medical history has six segments: chief complaint, history of present illness, past (medical) history, patient profile, family (medical) history, and review of systems (Table 1.2).

Chief Complaint

The chief complaint (CC) is the problem that the patient states precipitated this visit.

History of the Present Illness

The history of the present illness (HPI) is a narrative of the current problem(s). To clarify the **dimensions** or **parameters** of the patient's present illness, the following lines of questioning are followed:

Table 1.1
Process Guidelines for a Successful Medical Interview

Encouraging the narrative development
  Effective balance of open and closed questions
  Chronologic approach
Summarization
  For accuracy
  For acquiring additional information
Transition statements
Question types related to content area
  HPI: from open to closed
  PMH: closed and directive
  PP: from open to closed
  FH: closed
  ROS: closed
Effective closure of the interview
  Questions?
  Other concerns?
  Additions or corrections?
  Explain next step or finalize interaction

HPI, history of present illness; PHM, past medical history; PP, patient profile; FH, family (medical) history; ROS, review of systems.

- *Onset:* When did the patient first notice the symptom? What was he doing at the time?
- *Temporal sequence:* What has happened to the symptom since it was first noted? Has it gotten better or worse or remained the same? Has it become more or less frequent? How is it today compared with yesterday, or last week, or the time it first occurred? Has anything like this ever happened in the past? Are there any family members, coworkers, or friends with the same condition? (This is the framework of the narrative of the symptom. Effective methods for establishing this framework are detailed in the next section.)
- *Quality of the symptom:* What is it? Where in the body is it located? Does it move or radiate? How does it feel, look, smell, or sound?
- *Quantity of the symptom:* How bad or how extensive is the symptom? What words would the patient use to describe

Table 1.2
Content Components of the Medical History

Chief complaint (CC)	Patient profile (PP)
History of present illness (HPI)	Educational level
Onset	Occupational history
Temporal sequence or chronology	Current living situation
Quality of symptom(s)	Family structure and support
Quantity of symptom(s)	systems
Aggravating factors	Health habits
Alleviating factors	Diet and nutrition
Associated symptoms	Exercise
Contemporaneous medical	Tobacco, alcohol, and
problems	drug use
Past medical history (PHM)	Hobbies and special
Surgical procedures	interests
Other hospitalizations	Sexual activity and
Major trauma	concerns
Medications	Daily routine
Allergies	**Family (medical) history (FH)**
Childhood illnesses	**Review of systems (ROS)**
Immunization status	
Significant past medical illnesses	
Pregnancy and delivery history	

its quantity? On a scale of 1 (minimal) to 10 (agonizing), where would the patient place it?

- *Aggravating factors:* What, if anything, has been observed that will bring on the symptom or make it worse?
- *Alleviating factors:* What, if anything, has lessened the symptom or made it disappear? What has failed to do so? Has professional medical care been employed for this problem? What was done? Did it help? Have other remedies or treatments been attempted, such as over-the-counter drugs or nontraditional therapies?
- *Associated symptoms:* Has there been anything else different noticed by the patient or his associates? (This question is key to establishing symptom complexes or concurrent illness. When the patient's attention has been focused on a single symptom, there is commonly failure to mention others without specific prompting.) If the patient does have other symptoms, then connections between them are explored after each is characterized individually.

Past Medical History

The past medical history (PMH) is a catalog of significant past health problems. Significance represents a value judgment, so the assessment of what constitutes significant problems will vary from setting to setting and practitioner to practitioner. Problems you as the interviewer should always ask about include

- *Long-term past medical illnesses,* i.e., illnesses that have receded with treatment or on their own but that have potential for recurrence or late sequelae. Tuberculosis, certain malignancies (lymphoma or acute lymphocytic leukemia), hepatitis B, alcoholism, and severe depression, for example, fall into this category.
- *Surgical procedures,* i.e., any operation the patient has ever had, including the date of the operation, the symptoms that led to the procedure, the nature of the procedure, the final diagnosis, any adverse reactions to anesthesia (especially if additional surgery is contemplated), and any sequelae of the procedure.

- *Other hospitalizations,* i.e., the dates of, reasons for, and outcomes of the hospitalizations.
- *Major trauma not previously covered,* i.e., the nature of the trauma, the treatment rendered, and any resultant disability.
- *Medications,* i.e., all medications that are currently being taken or have been taken with any regularity in the past, including over-the-counter medications such as laxatives, aspirin, antihistamines, and vitamins, as patients seldom consider these nonprescription formulations as "medications" or "drugs" and therefore do not volunteer their use.
- *Allergies:* Seasonal, environmental, or food allergies along with their manifestations and treatments are documented. By far the most critical of these is any history of **medication allergies**. If a history of allergic reaction to any drug or agent used in diagnosis or treatment is obtained, the details of the reaction as well as the name of the substance involved should be ascertained. It is important to differentiate between true allergic reactions (e.g., skin rashes; histamine reactions such as facial and oral edema; allergic interstitial nephritis; or anaphylactic shock) and nonallergic side effects (e.g., nausea or loose stools). Because of the ubiquity of penicillin derivatives and the frequency of significant allergy to them, it is wise to ask specifically about penicillin reaction. An economical means of covering the ground is to ask, "Have you ever had an allergic reaction to penicillin or any other medicine?"
- *Childhood illnesses:* This information carries more importance in the history of a younger person than that of an older person. When the history indicates, elements to be included are common viral infections—mumps, rubella (German measles), rubeola (regular measles), chickenpox, and rheumatic fever.
- *Immunization status:* Essential data change with the age of the patient. All children and young adults should have a full immunization record for the chart, including immunization for measles, mumps, and rubella (MMR), hepatitis B, polio, diphtheria, pertussis, and tetanus (DPT, in children), and *Haemophilus influenzae* type B (HiB). Older adults and chronically ill patients of all ages

require annual influenza vaccine and immunization against pneumococcus once every 6 years. The date of the last tetanus shot should be ascertained.

* *Pregnancy and delivery history,* i.e., determination of the number of pregnancies, live births, and spontaneous or induced abortions, as well as documentation of types of delivery (vaginal or cesarean section) and any complications of pregnancies or deliveries.

Patient Profile

The patient profile (PP) is an inventory of medically relevant life-style. It is intended to give you as interviewer a sense of the patient as a member of society and of family and as a person who lives, works, and plays. The PP includes at a minimum

* *Educational level,* the highest attained.
* *Employment history,* current and past, with details of possible exposure to hazardous materials if relevant.
* *Current living situation,* including where and with whom.
* *Family structure and social support systems.*
* *Health habits,* including

    Diet: Number, content, and regularity of daily meals; food fads or special diets, such as vegetarianism, or unusual weight control diets.

    Exercise: Frequency and type of regular exercise.

    Tobacco use: Intensity of smoking is usually quantified as the number of packs of cigarettes smoked daily, multiplied by the number of years smoking, expressed as pack-years. If the patient no longer smokes, the same information is acquired, and the date of cessation is recorded. Pipe and cigar smoking require parallel documentation, as does the use of "smokeless" tobacco.

    Alcohol use: Type, amount, duration, and complications.

    Recreational drug use, such as cocaine, marijuana, or heroin, including type, frequency, duration, and complications.

* *Hobbies and special interests:* Modes of relaxation as well as clues to physical hazards or risks.

- *Sexual activity and/or concerns:* Extent and method are situation dependent. A good opening question might be, "Are you currently sexually active?" If the answer is no, ask, "Is this a problem for you?" Or, if the patient answers in the affirmative, a good next question is, "Have you any questions or concerns you would like to discuss?" If the patient has concerns and more detail is needed or if sexual practices are key to the HPI, extended questions and query techniques may be found under Extended (Problem-Focused) History and Physical Examination later in this chapter.

Family (Medical) History

The family (medical) history (FH) is a survey of the health of the patient's relatives and should include three generations: parents, siblings, and offspring, for the adult patient; and grandparents, parents, and siblings, for the child patient. For the elderly, inquiry about grandchildren yields more insight than questions about ancestors. The age and present state of health, including any significant disease, or age at death and cause of death should be ascertained for each pertinent family member. A secondary review is then made of any other history of potentially familial health problems, such as adult-onset diabetes mellitus, premature coronary heart disease or sudden unexpected death, cancer, high blood pressure, and Alzheimer's dementia.

Review of Systems

The review of systems (ROS) is a checklist usually reserved for the end of the interview and is designed as a final search for missed issues. This final check may bring to the surface a new and important problem. The list is a long series of closed questions. There are many variations on the content of the ROS available. One such list follows.

- *General:* Current weight and any recent change; fatigue; fever; energy level.

- *Endocrine:* History of thyroid disease; history of high blood sugar; recent intolerance to heat or cold; excessive thirst, hunger, or volume of urine output.
- *Hematologic:* History of anemia; easy bruising or difficulty controlling bleeding; history of blood transfusions including dates, reactions to blood products; history of blood clots or anticoagulation.
- *Psychiatric:* History of treatment for psychiatric or emotional problems; nervousness; anxiety; undue sadness; sleep disturbance; death wishes or suicidal thoughts.
- *Skin:* Recent changes in texture or appearance of hair, skin, or nails; new rashes, lumps, sores; history of treatment for skin condition.
- *Eyes:* Recent change in vision; blurring of vision; double vision; red or painful eyes; history of glaucoma or cataracts; most recent eye examination and results.
- *Nose and sinuses:* Increase in frequency of colds or nasal drainage; nosebleeds; history of sinus infections.
- *Mouth, throat, teeth:* Sores of tongue or mouth; dental problems and dental care history; bleeding of gums; hoarseness or voice change.
- *Neck:* Stiffness or injury; new lumps or swelling.
- *Breasts:* Tenderness; lumps; nipple discharge; history of self-examination; last physician examination and/or mammogram; any prior aspiration or biopsy.
- *Cardiorespiratory:* History of asthma, bronchitis, pneumonia, pleurisy, tuberculosis; new cough, sputum, coughing blood, wheezing, or shortness of breath. History of high blood pressure; heart disease; heart murmur; palpitations; chest pain; shortness of breath on exertion or while lying down; ankle swelling; history of electrocardiogram, chest x-ray, or other diagnostic tests.
- *Blood vessels:* Pain in legs with walking (how far); sensitivity or color change in fingers or toes with cold temperatures; varicose veins or history of phlebitis.
- *Gastrointestinal:* Difficulty swallowing, change in appetite; nausea, vomiting, diarrhea; abdominal pain, vomiting blood, or blood in stool; constipation or recent change in

bowel habits or appearance of stool; history of jaundice, liver or gallbladder problems; indigestion or new food intolerance.

- *Urinary:* Change in frequency of urination, volume of urine, or nature of stream; burning on urination; blood in urine; hesitancy; urgency; incontinence; history of urinary infections or stones; nocturia.
- *Male genitoreproductive:* History of hernia; venereal diseases; sores on penis; pain in testicle; frequency of testicular self-examination; sexual preference, function, satisfaction, or concerns if not raised and covered adequately in earlier portions of history.
- *Female genitoreproductive:* Menstrual history, including age of menarche, cycle length, pain with menses, change in duration, amount, or frequency of menses (may be omitted in the postmenopausal woman). For the older woman, history of age and any difficulty with menopause, such as hot flashes, irregular bleeding; history of hormone therapy, postmenopausal vaginal bleeding. For all postmenarchal women, history of venereal disease, vaginal discharge, painful sexual intercourse, vulvar itching, or unexpected vaginal bleeding. Sexual preference, activity, satisfaction, and concerns if they have not been discussed during other portions of the history. If not obtained earlier, the history of pregnancy and delivery, birth control method(s), and concerns about reproductive health may be asked at this time.
- *Musculoskeletal:* Muscle weakness, pain, tenderness, or stiffness; pain or swelling in joints; history of arthritis, gout, or back pain.
- *Neurologic:* History of headaches; seizures; blackouts; paralysis; numbness or tingling; trembling or weakness; difficulty speaking; memory loss or difficulty concentrating.

SCREENING (COMPREHENSIVE) PHYSICAL EXAMINATION

This outline for conducting a screening or comprehensive physical examination on an adult is sequenced to provide the greatest efficiency for you as examiner and the most comfort for the patient by minimizing position changes. The content is determined by consensus of the authors and published literature. Details may vary slightly from institution to institution (see Table 1.3).

The **four basic modes** applied to the physical examination are *inspection, palpation, percussion,* and *auscultation.* Each is used to varying degrees, depending on the body region being examined. The modes are defined as follows:

- *Inspection:* The inspection of the patient begins with general observation during the medical interview and is the pri-mary mode of the physical examination.
- *Palpation:* Light palpation is used to assess skin and superficial structures, variations in surface temperature,

Table 1.3
Examination Sequence

| Positions | | Examination | |
Patient	Examiner	Maneuver	Equipment
Seated	Facing patient	Inspect general appearance	
		Inspect hands	
		Palpate hands	
		Assess grip strength	
		Palpate radial pulse	
		Count radial pulse	Wristwatch
		Take blood pressure	Sphygmomano-meter, stethoscope
		Inspect scalp	
		Inspect face	
		Assess facial mobility and sensation	Cotton swab
		Inspect conjunctiva	
		Inspect sclera	
		Assess ocular movement	
		Assess visual fields	
		Assess hearing	

Table 1.3 *(continued)*
Examination Sequence

Positions		Examination	
Patient	Examiner	Maneuver	Equipment
		Assess pupillary reflexes	Penlight
		Funduscopic examination	Ophthalmo-scope
		Ear examination	Otoscope, speculum
		Inspect nose	Light, speculum
		Inspect oral cavity	Light, gauze, glove, tongue blade
		Assess deglutition	Cup of water
		Assess neck range of motion	
		Assess shoulder shrug, neck turning	
		Palpate head and neck lymph nodes	
		Inspect and palpate thyroid	
		Palpate carotid arteries	
Seated	Behind patient	Observe thorax and spine, posteriorly	
		Percuss spine for tenderness	
		Percuss costovertebral angle for tenderness	
		Test tactile fremitus, posterior lungs	
		Percuss posterior lungs	
		Auscult posterior lungs	Stethoscope
Seated	Facing patient	Auscult anterior and lateral lungs	Stethoscope
		Percuss anterior and lateral lungs	
		Inspect breasts	
		Palpate axillae	
Supine	To patient's right side	Palpate breast	
		Auscult precordium	Stethoscope
		Auscult carotid arteries	Stethoscope
		Inspect cervical veins	
		Observe abdomen	
		Auscult abdomen	Stethoscope

Table 1.3 *(continued)*
Examination Sequence

Positions		Examination	
Patient	Examiner	Maneuver	Equipment
		Percuss abdomen	
		Palpate liver	
		Palpate spleen	
		Palpate abdomen	
		Palpate inguinal lymph nodes	
		Palpate and auscult femoral arteries	Stethoscope
		Inspect and palpate legs and feet	
		Palpate leg and foot arteries	
		Test hip range of motion	
Seated	Facing patient	Test shoulder, elbow, knee, ankle range of motion	
		Test upper and lower limb muscle strength	
		Test muscle stretch reflexes	Percussion hammer
		Test plantar reflexes	Broken swab stick
		Test cerebellar function with rapid alternating motion and heel-to-shin tests	
		Test pain and light touch	Broken swab stick, cotton wisp
		Test vibratory sense, lower limbs	Tuning fork
Standing		Measure orthostatic pulse and blood pressure	Sphygmomanometer, stethoscope
Standing	Variable	Test back mobility	
		Test Romberg maneuver	
		Observe gait and transfers	
		Male genital and hernia examinations	Gloves
		Male rectal and prostate examinations	Gloves
Lithotomy		Female pelvic and rectal examination[a]	See Table 1.4

[a] Patients of either sex may be examined in the left lateral decubitus position.

moisture, or dryness. Deep palpation is applied to deep
visceral organs, such as those of the abdomen.

- *Percussion:* Use of sound to define structure, density, and
  content. The classical percussion method is to create
  vibration by tapping against the body surface, listening
  and feeling for differences in sound wave conduction.
- *Auscultation:* Use of the stethoscope to judge the movement of gases, fluids, or organs in body compartments.

Instruments and Supplies

The instruments and supplies listed in Table 1.4 include
everything used in doing the complete general examination.
The equipment of various specialists and subspecialists is not
included.

Table 1.4
Instruments and Supplies

Instruments	Supplies
Examining table	Examination gown
Thermometer	Half-sheet for draping
Sphygmomanometer	Disposable gloves
Stethoscope	Tongue blades
Ophthalmoscope	Paper cups
Otoscope	Cotton-tipped swabs
Penlight	Tape measure
Tuning fork(s)	Visual acuity chart of Snellen[a]
Percussion (reflex) hammer	Visual acuity chart, pocket
Nasal speculum or attachment	Gauze squares
Cloth measuring tape	Water-based lubricant gel
Paper and pencil	Stool occult-blood measure-
Wristwatch with sweep hand	ment card and developer
Skin-marking pencil	For pelvic examination
Equipment for measuring weight	Labeled glass slides
and height[a]	Papanicolaou devices for
Goose-neck lamp or other light	collecting cervical and
source[a]	endocervical cells
Vaginal speculum with light source	Fixative for slides

[a] Usually available in most clinical settings.

EXTENDED OR PROBLEM-FOCUSED EXAMINATION

EXTENDED (PROBLEM-FOCUSED) HISTORY AND PHYSICAL EXAMINATION

The extended (problem-focused) medical history is defined as a medical history concentrated exclusively on the immediate problem (present illness) and those elements from the other five segments of the screening history essential to understanding this single problem. Taking such a focused history requires a sound understanding of basic pathophysiology, hypothesis formulation, and information sorting, grounded in a knowledge of disease processes.

The expedience of providing care and the appropriate prioritization of patient needs are major demands dictating use of such a problem-directed assessment. Typical settings calling for the extended or problem-focused medical history are emergency rooms, immediate care centers, and ambulatory care sites.

The process of obtaining an extended (problem-focused) medical history differs from that utilized in the screening interview (Table 1.5). The clinician selects elements of the history essential to the solution, based on the nature and urgency of the problem at hand. The history is obtained in a modified order as well as in this abbreviated format.

In every medical history, certain "universal" data are collected: patient's age, occupation, current living situation, medications, and allergies.

In cases of an acute or exacerbated chronic situation, a confined symptom related to a single physiologic system, or planned follow-up on a specific complaint with which the patient presents to office or emergency department, the interview follows the general principles tabulated above and focuses on the information needed to solve the problem identified by the patient as the purpose for the visit.

A second type of focused medical history may be indicated when preliminary questioning in the screening interview raises concerns for either patient or provider that a problem may exist. Specific content areas in which an expanded history is needed are developed below. Included are *(a)* the indications for the focus and *(b)* questioning details to facilitate information collection.

Table 1.5
Process of Focused History Acquisition

Step	Comment
1. Elicit CC	CC provides entry into the immediate problem
2. Obtain HPI, including the seven dimensions of the symptom(s) Onset Chronology Quality Quantity Aggravating factors Alleviating factors Associated symptoms	Obtain this information in precisely the way it is pursued in the screening history
3. Hypothesis formulation	This primary formulation will guide the clinician to the systems needing review (selected ROS)
4. Collect pertinent ROS data, both positives and negatives	Select the systems to be reviewed based on the primary diagnostic hypotheses
5. Hypothesis modulation	With new information, modify diagnostic considerations if necessary
6. Do selective FH, PMH, and PP	Content of FH, PMH, and PP is dictated by the working hypotheses
7. Refine	With the primary data collected, now reprioritize diagnostic hypotheses
8. Test hypotheses	Plan the segments of the focused physical examination to be done in order to test the diagnostic hypotheses generated by the history

Extended Sexual History

INDICATIONS FOR AN EXTENDED SEXUAL HISTORY

1. A chief complaint or history of present illness clearly or possibly relating to sexual activity
2. A specific question or concern about sexual function raised by the patient
3. A clinician's concern that sexual function or behavior patterns may contribute to the patient's symptom(s)
4. An unexpected finding on physical examination that suggests that more information about the patient's sexual function or behavior patterns is needed

A nonjudgmental, openly inquiring attitude is imperative to successful acquisition of sexual information. Assume nothing. Never show surprise. Sexual practices are so diverse that you cannot predict them accurately. For example, gender preferences are often pertinent to understanding the patient's medical problems; they must be discovered but never judged. Stereotypic models of preference and behavior patterns have no place in the medical encounter. Ask fully open-ended questions and allow the patient to describe sexual practices in his own way. Save specific or closed questions for follow-up or areas not covered thereby.

SEXUAL ISSUES RAISED BY THE HISTORY OF PRESENT ILLNESS

When the chief complaint or present illness suggests sexual issues, follow necessary leads in developing the extended history, e.g., with acute or chronic abdominal pain, penile or vaginal discharge, dysuria or urinary incontinence, secondary amenorrhea, change in pattern of menstrual bleeding, undesired infertility, dyspareunia. Clinicians must remain aware of the potential relationship between the patient's presenting problem and sexual practices. When an extended sexual history is thus indicated, ask the following questions:

- Number of sexual partners and nature of encounters
  1. Is there a single partner? Multiple partners?
  2. What is the gender of each partner?
  3. What has been the frequency of recent intimate sexual contacts?

4. How much does the patient know about the health of the recent contacts?
5. Does the patient regularly practice "safer sex?" What protective methods are used?

- Nature of sexual practices
    1. What types of intercourse does the patient engage in: vaginal, anal, oral, or combinations?
    2. Does the patient use sexual aid devices (apparatus) with a partner? Alone? If so, what are the specifics?
    3. Does the patient use lubricants, spermicides, scented products? Are there other hygienic practices, such as immediate postcoital voiding or douching?
    4. Are there any other details of sexual practices that the patient is willing to supply?

SPECIFIC SEXUAL CONCERNS RAISED BY THE PATIENT

During the interview, the patient may have specific questions or concerns about personal sexual function. Below are some questions that the clinician may employ.

Sexual Concerns Specific to Men

Impotence. It is important to define what a man means by the word, i.e., inability to attain and maintain an erection long enough for intromission? Loss of sexual desire? Anorgasmia? Inability to ejaculate? Premature ejaculation? Ask the following questions:

1. How often and under what specific circumstances is the patient unable to attain (or maintain) penile erection?
2. How long has the problem been present?
3. Is it getting better, worse, or not changing?
4. Is he able to masturbate to erection?
5. Does he awaken with erection?
6. Is he taking any medications or recreational drugs? If so, what are the names, doses, and temporal relation ship to impotence?
7. How much alcohol does he use?
8. Does he have any known chronic illness?

9. Are there concurrent stresses in the patient's life, particularly in his relationship(s) with his sexual partner(s)?
10. Are there symptoms of aortic vascular insufficiency (e.g., buttock claudication)?
11. Has the man sired a child in the past (establishes prior function)?
12. Is there a history of diabetes mellitus?
13. Is libido preserved or lost?

Sexual Concerns Common to Men and Women

Loss of libido (sexual desire). Determine the specifics.
1. What is the chronology of the complaint?
2. Is it partner-specific?
3. Are there stresses in the relationship(s), sexual or otherwise?
4. Are there other life stresses?
5. Does the general medical history raise other health problems as the potential basis for loss of sexual interest?
6. Are there signs and symptoms of depression?

Lack of sexual responsiveness. This is frequently referred to by the patient or partner as "frigidity." Try to determine the following:
1. Precisely what does the patient experience that is being regarded as lack of responsiveness? Lack of interest in sex? If so, the clinician pursues the same line of questioning as outlined for the patient describing loss of desire. Or is it fear of pregnancy or sexually transmitted disease, experience of pain with intercourse, unacceptable sexual practices, emotional reaction to prior unpleasant or brutal sexual encounter, or fear of precipitating or suffering stroke, heart attack, or sudden death?
2. What are the details of past and current sexual practices and dissatisfactions?

Sexual Concerns Specific to Women

Anorgasmia. This refers to the inability to achieve orgasm. Try to determine the specific type:

1. Has the patient ever achieved orgasm, either with masturbation or with a partner?
2. Does the patient achieve orgasm under certain circumstances (what are they?) and not under others (what are they?)?
3. Is she erratically and unpredictably unable to have an orgasm (random anorgasmia)?
4. What is the chronology of the anorgasmia, and can it be related by history to physical, pharmacologic, emotional, social, or interpersonal events?

Dyspareunia. This refers to pain or discomfort on intercourse. Determine the following:

1. What are the details of the complaint, e.g., the location, nature, and duration of the pain, the timing of the pain relative to the sequence of the sexual act (on intromission, with deep thrusting, postcoital, etc.), the relationship of pain to body position during intercourse?
2. Is it new or longstanding? Partner-specific? Cyclic, related to the menstrual cycle? To bowel function? To voiding? Getting better, worse, or unchanged? Are there alleviating or aggravating factors?
3. Does the patient feel she has adequate vaginal lubrication prior to intromission? If not, have lubricants been used, and if so, what is the effect?
4. Is she satisfied with the nonsexual aspects of the relationship(s) with her partner(s)?
5. What are the details of sexual practices, such as use of devices that might be causing perineal or vaginal trauma?
6. Has the patient ever been a victim of rape or other sexual violence?
7. Is the patient able to supply any insights into the cause of the painful intercourse?

8. Is there postcoital vaginal bleeding or spotting (important both for diagnosis and for affective context)?

SEXUAL CONCERNS RAISED BY PHYSICAL EXAMINATION

Common findings that suggest the need for an extended sexual history are

- Signs of genital, perianal, perineal, or oral trauma
  Bruises
  Excoriations
  Bites
  Tears
- Evidence of infection
  Urethral or vaginal discharge
  Condyloma
  Inguinal or generalized lymphadenopathy
  Pubic lice
  Genital vesicles
- Unexplained pelvic tenderness or mass
- Cervical abnormalities
  Friability
  Discharge
  Pain on motion
- Vaginal atrophy or vulvovaginitis

Extended Substance Use History

It is your responsibility as clinician to seek details of substance use when there is any suggestion of a problem. This realm requires sensitivity to the possibility of denial as well as a nonjudgmental approach. Alcohol, since it is the drug most commonly used—and abused—in our society, will be dealt with separately from other chemicals, such as marijuana, cocaine, and heroin.

Alcohol, because it is legal, readily available, and an intrinsic part of our social lives, presents particular hazards for the consumer. It is your responsibility as clinician to assess drinking patterns in each patient for whom you are responsible.

If the answers to one or more are positive or if the affective nonverbal responses are suggestive, the clinician should have a follow-up. Morning drinking has a very high predictive value for alcoholism. The typical patient with an alcohol problem will not discuss his drinking based on denial, cognitive deficits, and/or painful feelings of anxiety, guilt, and shame. These are difficult to overcome. Try the following strategy:

1. Focus on the *effects* of alcohol consumption rather than on frequency and quantity. "What happens when you drink?" Whether addicted or not, people with alcohol problems drink when they do not intend to, drink more than they intend to, and suffer some mixture of emotional, physical, social, occupational, financial, and legal difficulty when they drink uncontrollably. Ask, "Have you ever been arrested for driving under the influence of alcohol?"

2. Maintain an accepting attitude of the patient as person while discussing his drinking patterns ("love the sinner, hate the sin"). Low self-esteem is common in alcoholics. Positive reinforcement of good qualities will greatly facilitate the interview and the therapeutic alliance.

3. As rapport is established, persist in direct questioning. Ask about alcohol and withdrawal-related physical symptoms, such as blackouts, shakiness, or seizures. Explore conflicts and regrets about drinking. Inquire about family, job problems, and legal problems, especially difficulties with DWI (driving while intoxicated) or DUI (driving under the influence). Ask directly about depression and suicidal ideation.

Other than alcohol, the most frequently used substances in the United States are **marijuana, cocaine, amphetamines,** and **heroin.** The legal problems of use of these substances add another dimension to the difficulty of getting accurate information. A nonjudgmental approach will facilitate data collection.

When a patient acknowledges that he uses any of these substances, inquire about the method of use. For example, are amphetamines taken by mouth or intravenously? In what form(s) and by what route(s) is cocaine taken? Additional questions might include the following:

1. Do you use more than one substance at a time?
2. Are you always able to stop using when you want to?
3. Have you had "flashbacks" or "blackouts" as a result of using?
4. Do others express concern about your substance use?
5. Do you ever feel guilty about using?
6. Have you experienced withdrawal symptoms when you've stopped using, or have you been treated to prevent withdrawal symptoms?
7. Have you had medical problems as a result of using, such as convulsions, heart or skin infections, venous clots, memory loss, hepatitis, or a positive HIV test?
8. Have you missed work or lost a job because of using?
9. How do you get the money to purchase the substance(s)?
10. Have you been in trouble with the law as a result of using?
11. Do you skin-pop (a method of injecting drugs that is utilized when there are no longer usable veins)?
12. Do you shoot the pocket? (This is an injection—often by a paid assistant—of the junction of the internal jugular and subclavian veins and is fraught with medical complications.)
13. Do you share needles? Do you clean them?
14. How do you clean your "works?"
15. What water source do you use to dilute (tap, toilet, etc.)?
16. Have you been in any addiction-treatment programs?

If any of the questions is answered in the affirmative, ask the patient to provide details.

Focused Family Violence History

Abuse of children, spouses, or the elderly is estimated to occur in a quarter of American families. Prepare to pursue this possibility, particularly in the setting of suspicious injuries. A nonjudgmental attitude is essential for getting optimal information.

When suspicion is raised by trauma as the presenting complaint, the inquiry should be direct. "Tell me exactly what happened when you fell down the stairs." If the response does not make sense or does not correlate with the injuries sustained or the patient is evasive or vague, be more explicit. "Were you pushed by someone?" Persistence in acquiring details of an injury may overcome defenses.

If the patient initially denies abuse, the topic can be raised again as a part of the personal profile: "Who lives in your household?" "How are relationships among members of the household?" "How do you resolve disagreements?" "Does anyone ever hit you?"

Family history provides another opportunity to explore the possibility of violence. "Was your mother beaten by your father?" "Were you or your spouse abused as children?" A "yes" mandates a return to the presenting injury complaint and to abuse questions. Also ask

1. Have bones ever been broken?
2. Does sexual abuse take place along with physical abuse?
3. Have burns, punctures, slashing, whipping, or confining been practiced?
4. What other person has been victimized by the same abuser?
5. Has legal action, such as a restraining order, ever been implemented?
6. Has help ever been received from social agencies or from a victims' assistance group?
7. Is the abuser likely to remain in the household (or visit the health care site), and what is the potential for further violence?

Focused Mental Health History

Vestiges of our cultural nonacceptance of emotional distress sometimes make the mental health history a difficult content area in the medical interview. Clues that a detailed mental health history should be pursued include

1. Presenting symptoms that are commonly associated with emotional disturbance, e.g., recent changes in weight, difficulty sleeping, trouble concentrating, memory impairment, fatigue

2. Feelings of worthlessness or hopelessness
3. A history of current substance use
4. A history of recent major change in family or job status
5. A family history of mental illness
6. A history of prior treatment for emotional problems
7. Accelerated or sustained high stress in the patient's environment
8. Chronic illness, disability, or a newly diagnosed serious illness
9. Inappropriate affect—blunted or exaggerated—during the interview
10. Poor personal hygiene or negligence in dress, or extravagant, inappropriately formal, elegant attire
11. Evidence of a thought disorder, difficulty remembering details of the medical history, or an inability to engage in normal conversation

Initial questions should be open-ended and phrased so as not to cause defensiveness. "How has your mood been?" "How are you sleeping?" "How is your energy?" More detailed, closed questioning must always include questions about *prescription and over-the-counter medications.*

Symptoms suggestive of *depression* or situations that the patient perceives as hopeless demand a determination of *suicide risk.* The best way to approach the potential for suicide is by direct questions: "Do you ever think about killing yourself?" "Do you ever wish you were dead?" If the answer is "yes," follow with the question, "Have you thought about how you would kill yourself?" Ask the patient to describe his plan, then determine whether he has means available, and ask, "Would you go through with it?" Inquire about any past attempts at suicide. The patient at risk for suicide constitutes a medical emergency and should not be allowed to leave the premises. Immediate psychiatric consultation is imperative. Elderly men have the highest ratio of completed to attempted suicide. Adolescents and the aged often present atypically, with a less dysphoric depression.

Focused Environmental Health History

Because hazardous exposures may cause nondiagnostic symptoms involving any body system and may mimic more ordinary medical diseases, the following points should be incorporated into the screening medical history:

1. Obtain in the HPI any temporal relationship to work or home activities, any history (recent or remote) of toxic exposure, and contributing factors such as smoking or medications. An illness similar in description to that of the patient in a family member or work colleague may reflect *(a)* a true common exposure (toxic or infective), *(b)* the psychologic tendency to develop or recognize symptoms that an associate has, or *(c)* mere coincidence.
2. Obtain a full employment history, current and remote, with information about duties. Include work done during military service.
3. Remember that *recreation* as well as occupation can produce these exposures (e.g., a hobby involving soldering of lead).

When there appears to be a relationship between symptoms and setting, further explore the potential sources.

Work exposure. Obtain the following information:

1. A full list of all jobs held, with the description of duties, duration, and dates
2. A full list of sites of employment and products manufactured
3. A full account of the worker's tasks at each job and, if available, diagnoses
4. A description of any similar symptoms among fellow workers
5. An account of what protective measures were employed, such as noise protection, ear guards, ventilation, lead aprons, respirators, and gloves, and how consistently the individual employed them
6. An account of any monitoring that was done of personal (radiation badges, serial chest radiographs, etc.) or work site (measurements on air, water)

Other environmental exposure. Obtain the following information:

1. A description of neighborhood pollution, such as nearby industry, exposure to contaminated work clothes of other family members (a recognized mechanism of asbestosis in spouses of insulation workers), and sickness among neighbors
2. A description of possible exposure to household toxins, such as pesticides, chemicals used in hobbies, aerosols, cleaning fluids, or disinfectants, and information about ventilation when using potentially hazardous chemicals and symptoms manifested by any family member

Follow-up information. If any of the other questions yield positive answers, ask about

1. The product or the chemical composition of any suspected or possibly harmful substance to which the patient has been or is exposed
2. The physical form used, e.g., liquid, dust or powder, or gas
3. How the substance is handled, e.g., the protective measures used, operating and cleanup procedures, surveillance procedures, ventilation of the area
4. The potential mode of entry of the substance, e.g., skin exposure, inhalation, eating or smoking with contaminated hands

Focused Dietary and Nutritional History

INDICATIONS FOR EXTENDING THE DIETARY HISTORY

Symptoms Elicited in the History of Present Illness

Symptoms elicited in the HPI that are indications for extending the dietary history include

1. Recent loss or gain of more than 10% of previous weight
2. Presence of a chronic disease, such as diabetes mellitus, gastrointestinal disease, hyperlipidemia, vascular disease, or hypertension

3. A condition that increases metabolic demands, such as protracted infection, trauma, malignancy, burns, or bedsores
4. A condition in which nutrient losses are increased, such as vomiting, diarrhea, chronic blood loss, hemodialysis, or draining sites of infection
5. A change in the ability to cut and handle food, to chew, or to swallow
6. Residence in a nursing home coupled with any of the above
7. Concerns specifically raised by the patient or care givers

Concerns Raised by Clues in Other Portions of the Screening History

Concerns raised by clues in other portions of the screening history that are indications for extending the dietary history include

1. A PMH of food allergies or intolerances
2. A history of difficulty adhering to prior diets prescribed for medical conditions
3. A history of fad or crash dieting, use of appetite depressants or stimulants
4. A FH of diseases that may genetically predispose the patient to nutritional risk, e.g., diabetes mellitus, breast or colon cancer, hyperlipidemia
5. PP indicators that the patient's life-style may place him at risk for nutritional disorders, e.g., alcohol consumption, limited finances, physical disability that may impair food shopping or preparation, or ethnic or cultural food practices that are difficult to follow in the patient's microenvironment

Signs From the Physical Examination

Signs from the physical examination that are indications for extending the dietary history include

1. Body weight varying more than 20% from ideal

2. Unexplained skin or mucous membrane abnormalities, such as angular cheilosis, gingival bleeding, glossitis, or diffuse rashes
3. Extensive dental caries, particularly on the posterior (lingual) aspect of teeth
4. Subcutaneous or tendinous nodular deposits suggesting xanthomas
5. Poor muscle development and/or tone that is not otherwise explicable

Abnormalities on Laboratory Testing, Such as Unexpected Lymphopenia or Hypoalbuminemia

If it is determined that a detailed nutritional history is necessary, several areas may be developed.

A 24-hour dietary recall. Ask the patient to recite in detail what he ate during the past 24 hours. Each meal is described in terms of what foods, what quantities, and how frequently the patient ate. Was this day's food intake typical?

A history of dietary additives. Does the patient take vitamins or food supplements? If so, which ones and what quantities does he take each day? For how long has he supplemented his diet? Does he use laxatives? If so, what type and how often?

A history of dietary aversions or taboos. What types of foods does the patient never eat?

Current use of any prescription or over-the-counter medications. Does the patient take any "medications" that could lead to a nutrient-drug interaction?

Attitude toward eating and toward dietary habits. Does he enjoy food? Does he snack or rely on "fast food" for nutrition? Can he taste and smell his food? Has there been any change in appetite? Does the patient worry about being too thin or too fat? If so, how does he address the problem?

Nutritional resources. Does the patient have the financial and physical resources—including teeth—to maintain adequate nutrition? Does he possess an understanding of healthy dietary habits?

If you are suspicious of any problems with nutrition but are unable to gain adequate information from these queries, you may choose to ask the patient to keep a written food diary (quantitative and qualitative) for several days. Alternatively, the patient may be referred to a nutritionist for assessment.

HIV History

The rapidly evolving understanding of HIV disease mandates that this section be considered provisional. The extended history currently related to HIV infection is indicated for risk assessment *(a)* when the patient expresses concerns about exposure, *(b)* when the clinician discovers suspicious abnormalities on physical examination, and *(c)*, in modified form, when a patient with known HIV disease is seen.

Risk assessment. To determine risk for HIV, ask about
1. Sexual history (see extended sexual history).
2. An intravenous and/or parenteral drug use history including time frame, frequency, and sharing of apparatus (see Extended Substance Use History).
3. A history of blood product transfusions. What products were received? When and where? Essentially all blood products in the United States since 1985–1986 have been safe. Prior exposures or exposures in other locales represent higher risk.

Occupational exposure is relatively unlikely. However, inquire about whether the patient has been involved in handling bodily secretions of HIV-positive patients? If so, were there needle-stick injuries or splashes onto open wounds, dermatitic skin, or mucosal surfaces (eyes, mouth).

Patient concerns. If a patient expresses concerns that he may have been exposed to HIV, ask him why. Inquire about any information missing from the risk assessment history. A history of no high-risk behavior coupled with persistent or major concerns may reflect any of four situations:
1. Ignorance about transmission
2. Susceptibility to popular hysterical attitudes toward HIV
3. An incomplete database, often resulting from reticence or concealment about risky behavior
4. Psychologic disturbance, a gamut from heightened and global anxiety to frank delusions of AIDS

Unexplained physical findings. Very few findings are specific for HIV disease, but be alert to the possibility if there is unexplained

1. Generalized lymphadenopathy
2. Retinal abnormalities, particularly cotton-wool spots in an otherwise-healthy young person, or the unexplained combination of retinal exudates and hemorrhages coursing along the retinal vessels
3. Mental status abnormalities, most specifically evidence of cognitive impairment without psychopathology in a young person
4. Kaposi's sarcoma (KS) of skin (KS of the feet or lower legs in elderly men of Jewish or Mediterranean descent does not increase suspicion of HIV disease) or of mouth or strikingly severe psoriasis, seborrheic dermatitis, or polydermatomal bilateral herpes zoster infection
5. Fever that is protracted and unexplained by history
6. Stool samples positive for blood, if otherwise unexplained
7. Severe, extraordinary, necrotic and ulcerative genital and/or oral herpes simples lesions
8. Unexplained oral lesions of thrush, any hairy leukoplakia, or KS

Patient with known HIV disease. Since HIV typically causes a chronic and progressive fatal illness, consider

- *Functional status and activities of daily living:* How many of the required activities of daily living is the patient able to carry out for himself? Does he have the physical and financial assistance he needs? What additional services would enhance his quality of life? Who is doing the laundry? Shopping? Food preparation? Cleaning of home? Administration of medications?
- *Support systems:* Are emotional and social needs being met? Does he have a support network adequate to provide comfort and companionship? Is he in touch with special service organizations?
- *Nutrition:* Inanition is often a major problem. In addition, adverse reactions to medications commonly cause nausea,

so the potential for being weakened through malnutrition is commonly amplified.

- *Bowel function:* Refractory diarrhea occurs frequently in patients with AIDS, sometimes from infections or enteric neoplasia, sometimes from medicines, sometimes from HIV itself, and sometimes from treatment. Find out about its presence and severity.

- *Preventive therapy and immunizations:* Many patients with AIDS receive pills (such as zidovudine), monthly inhalations of pentamidine, and often a host of other treatments. Review these to ascertain supply, cost, consistency of use, and problems. This is also a good time to review, if necessary, the patient's awareness and practice regarding transmission of HIV to others, in particular via needles, blood products, and sex, and nontransmission via social contact and ordinary activities of daily living.

- *Cough, respiratory status, and supplemental oxygen:* Respiratory difficulties may dominate symptoms in AIDS.

- *Pain control:* The presence, locale, and severity of pain depend on particular complications. Inquiry establishes information and enhances empathy.

- *Mouth care:* Some oral complications such as pernicious gingivitis can be minimized with good oral hygiene, so the effort of asking and counseling is well justified.

- *Visual function:* Cytomegalovirus retinitis can cause blindness, so ask about its earliest symptoms in AIDS—visual floaters, reduced visual acuity, and visual field cuts.

- *Nontraditional and unproven therapies:* Have the patient fill you in on herbal medicines or other products he is using that are unapproved.

- *Advance directives:* Many persons with AIDS will have strong preferences about feeding tubes, CPR, and the use of mechanical ventilation. **The routine visit is the time to establish these, not when an acute crisis occurs**.

- *Coping with impending death:* What are his fears and concerns about the immediate and the distant future? What plans has he made for dealing with difficulties as they arise? Who does he call in an emergency? When he needs to talk or cry?

2

General Appearance and Vital Signs

GENERAL APPEARANCE

Goals. Collect the most basic information about functional state, diagnoses, and severity of illness early in the clinical encounter.

Technique. Look at the patient, top to bottom.

Interpretation. Among the issues to be interpreted are acuity of illness and the toxic state; deformities and asymmetries; large skin lesions; distinguishing between physical and psychic distress (often impossible); mobility, both overall and of major body regions; states of nutrition and hydration (see Tables 2.1–2.3).

Table 2.1
Principal Specific Diagnoses Often Best Made on General Appearance

Depression
Hypothyroidism
Hyperthyroidism
Acromegaly
Scleroderma

Table 2.2
Major Causes of Looking Younger Than Stated Age

Intentional misreport
Transcription or recording error
Cosmetic use and cosmetic surgery
Obesity
Local facial edema
Systemic sclerosis
Corticosteroid therapy
Immunosuppressive therapy, other therapy
Anorexia nervosa

Table 2.3
Major Causes of Looking Older Than Stated Age

Intentional misreport
Transcription or recording error
Cigarette smoking
Excess **solar exposure**
Severe underweight
Morbid obesity
Chronic illness
Marked fatigue
Psychiatric illness
Widespread arterial disease

Table 2.4
Principal Palpable Pulses in Most Healthy Adults[a], from Head to Toe

Superficial temporal artery anterior to ear
Superior orbital artery, near 12 o'clock position on orbital rim[a]
Common carotid artery in mid to upper lateral neck
Subclavian artery behind junction of middle and medial thirds of clavicle[a]
Aortic arch inferoposterior to sternal notch[a]
Cardiac apex[a]
Brachial artery under biceps tendon
Radial artery at wrist
Ulnar artery[a]
Digital arteries on ulnar aspects of fingers, especially second, third, and fourth fingers at or about proximal interphalangeal joints[a]
Abdominal aorta in epigastrium or just below[a]
Femoral artery at inguinal ligament
Popliteal artery in popliteal fossa[a]
Dorsalis pedis artery at some point(s) between extensor retinaculum of foot and hallux-second toe interspace[a]
Posterior tibial artery, 1 fingerbreadth behind medial malleolus

[a] Palpable only in about one-half of normal adults.

VITAL SIGNS

The **vital signs** are **pulse, respiration, temperature,** and **blood pressure.** All should be measured in every complete examination and in many briefer encounters. They are vital because they are quantitative clinical measurements of enormous value.

Pulse

Goals. Determine the rate and regularity of cardiac action and the state of arterial flow.

Technique. Touch and count pulsatile skin overlying arteries, most commonly the radial artery (Tables 2.4 and 2.5). Once you have found a pulse, "park" there to assess rate, regularity of both timing and force, intensity, and character.

Interpretation. In normal adults, a rate of 50–100 beats/minute is expected (Table 2.6).

PULSE PRESSURE

Pulse pressure is the palpable force of pulsation, the difference between the systolic and the diastolic pressure. Normal pulse pressure in healthy adults ranges from 30 to 70 torr.

PULSUS PARADOXUS

Pulsus paradoxus is an exaggeration of the normal (0–8 torr) decrease in systolic blood pressure (SBP) and, thus, in pulse pressure, on inspiration. When you feel the pulse weaken on inspiration, the drop must be 20 torr or more.

Table 2.5
Measures to Find the Radial Pulse

Try the other side
Try *passively* flexing the wrist a few degrees
Try moving a bit proximally
Move a bit distally
Lighten the pressure
Intensify the pressure if lightening the pressure fails

Table 2.6
Principal Causes of Sinus Bradycardia (Regular Rate Below 50/minute)

Normal finding in some trained athletes
Idioventricular rhythm and other lower pacemakers
Intrinsic disease of the cardiac conduction system, e.g., sick sinus syndrome
Medications, e.g., β-blockers, digoxin
Extreme hyperbilirubinemia

Slow, quiet breathing is essential to render a pulsus para-doxus perceptible.

Respirations

Goals. Determine the speed of breathing to assess cardiopulmonary and neurologic integrity and function (Table 2.7).

Technique. Stand behind the patient and, without his knowing, observe his chest cage. An alternative technique is to auscultate over the upper sternum (not trachea) but tell the patient you are counting heartbeats. Count for 15 seconds if

Table 2.7
Principal Causes of Respiratory Distress (Observed With General Appearance or While Counting Respirations)

Cardiac dysfunction, particularly on the left side of the heart; most commonly, the left ventricle
Pulmonary disease
Extrapulmonary respiratory problems (nares, nasopharynx, larynx, trachea)
Acidosis
Anxiety and panic

the rate and regularity are normal and for a longer time if they are abnormal.

Interpretation. A normal respiratory rate is 12–18 cycles/minute in healthy young and middle-aged adults and somewhat faster in healthy aged persons. A normal respiratory rate does not mean that oxygenation is adequate. Chronic obstructive pulmonary disease and narcotic drugs can slow both chemosensing and response. Anxiety speeds up respiration, as do other psychologic stimuli.

Temperature Measurement

Goals. Determine normality, fever, and hypothermia.

Technique. *Shake down* all mercury thermometers to 35°C (95°F) or below before inserting. After 4 minutes, remove and inspect the thermometer without shaking down.

- **Oral (blue-tipped):** Instruct the patient to avoid clamping teeth on instrument, which is placed sublingually.

- *Rectal (red-tipped):* A small amount of Vaseline may be applied over the bulb (low-number) end of the instrument and smeared one-third up the outside of the thermometer. Then the thermometer is gently inserted 4 cm into the rectum toward the patient's navel and is left in this position for 4 minutes.
- *Axillary:* The thermometer is placed in the axilla with the ipsilateral arm passively adducted and immobilized to cover it.
- *Electronic:* The probe, enclosed in a sterile disposable sheath, is placed under the patient's tongue and is left in place until completion is indicated electronically.
- *Ear probes (infrared tympanic membrane measurements):* Follow the manufacturer's directions for their use.

Interpretation. In normal adults, oral temperatures typically range between 36°C and 37.5°C, with late afternoon and evening temperatures exceeding those taken earlier in the day, sometimes by as much as 1°C. Axillary temperatures are lowest and least accurate. Oral temperatures are next higher. Rectal temperatures are the highest of all and most accurate, with evening rectal temperatures ranging up to 37.8°C in many normal persons. Tympanic measurements are plagued by false elevations with no consistent correction factor. For more interpretation, see Tables 2.8–2.11.

Rapid breathing lowers oral temperatures, as does mouth breathing. The drinking of hot liquids can produce false elevations; the drinking of cold liquids can artificially lower the reading.

Beware of intentional falsification! Measuring the temperature of freshly voided urine with an electronic device can "end-run" this problem.

Blood Pressure Measurement

Goals. Determine the presence of normotension, hypertension, or hypotension; further assess cardiovascular function, vascular flow, and intravascular volume status.

Technique. Blood pressure (BP) measurement is complex; see Details of the technique, which follows.

Table 2.8
Major Causes of Fever

Infections of all types
Ovulation
Luteal phase of menstrual cycle
Pregnancy
Medications, e.g., tricyclic antidepressants, neuroleptics, other
  agents with antimuscarinic properties, progesterone
Central fever from brain/brainstem dysfunction
Biologic agents, e.g., therapeutic interleukins and interferons
Environmental heat exposure
Surgery (including when not complicated by infection)
Tissue necrosis, e.g., myocardial infarction
Factitious fever
Vasculitides
Other inflammatory disorders, e.g., ulcerative colitis
Malignancies, particularly lymphoma, leukemia, renal cell carcinoma,
  hepatocellular carcinoma, or liver metastases from any cancer
Pulmonary embolism
Deep venous thrombosis
Thyrotoxicosis, particularly thyroid storm; rarely, Addisonism
?Psychologic stress
?Intravascular **volume depletion**
Fecal impaction

Table 2.9
Principal Causes of Fever Without Tachycardia

Legionella infection
Salmonella infection, especially typhoid fever
Ornithosis ("psittacosis")
Drug-induced fever, especially **drug fever** (allergic)
Factitious fever
Sinoatrial node dysfunction, pharmacogenic (digoxin, β–blockade)
  or native, i.e., underlying problems of cardiac automaticity and
  response, either structural or functional (e.g., extreme hyper-
  bilirubinemia)

Details of the technique.
1. Eliminate extraneous sound while auscultating: Turn off the television, close the door, turn off monitors, and request interruption of all nearby speech.
2. Remove any garment that covers or constricts the patient's upper arm.

Table 2.10
Principal Causes of Extreme Pyrexia (Fever Above 40.5°C)

Infection
Autonomic failure producing **central fever**
Neuroleptic malignant syndrome
Severe environmental **exposure** (extreme heat wave, unventi-
  lated and un-air-conditioned environments), with or without
  sunstroke/heatstroke
Drug-related fevers, especially with defective heat dissipation
  due to antimuscarinic drug actions
Malignant hyperthermia (specific entity after certain anesthetics)

Table 2.11
Fever in the Critical Care Unit

Infection	Tissue necrosis
Pneumonia	**Myocardial infarction**
Septicemia and infections associated with foreign bodies such as intravascular catheters	Hepatic infarct
	Multiorgan failure
Other	Central fever
Drug fever	**Blood transfusion reaction**
	Venous thrombosis and pulmonary embolism

3. Have the patient sit quietly for 5 minutes in a room with comfortable ambient temperature.
4. Palpate the patient's brachial pulse.
5. Apply the sphygmomanometer with the distal edge of the cuff 1.5 cm proximal to the brachial pulse.
6. Lock the release valve.
7. Inflate the cuff while palpating the radial pulse.
8. Pulsation will become faint, then impalpable, as the dial rises. This is near the SBP. Open the valve slightly so pressure drops about 3 torr/second.
9. When the pulse becomes palpable again, note the dial reading. This is the *SBP by palpation.*
10. Deflate the cuff and wait 15 seconds.
11. In the meantime, place the diaphragm of the stethoscope directly on the *brachial* pulse site.

12. Close the valve tightly. Reinflate the instrument to 20 torr above the SBP that was measured by palpation.
13. Start listening through the stethoscope.
14. Open the valve so that the cuff pressure drops by 3 torr/second.
15. The point at which you first hear faint tapping (**Korotkoff sound** I) is the SBP (by auscultation).
16. The intensity of Korotkoff sounds will increase as the cuff pressure falls.
17. As cuff pressure falls further, the sounds muffle, defining phase IV, and then disappear, defining phase V.
18. Record phase V as the *diastolic blood pressure* (DBP).

In patients whose Korotkoff sounds muffle (phase IV) but never disappear completely (phase V), record phases I, IV, and V together—a practice otherwise unnecessary— as, for instance, 130/75/0.

Interpretation. In normal adults, the BP measurements tend to range between 90/60 and 140/90. Below this is hypotension and above this is hypertension. All readings are interpreted in light of a particular patient's prior BP. The BP normally fluctuates widely for many reasons, including time of day, most recent meal, etc.

Discrepant side-to-side readings. If there is a discrepancy between BPs in the arms, use the arm with the higher reading. If the leg must be used, recall that in the normal adult, SBP usually measures 20–30 torr higher in the leg than in the arm, whereas DBP may be unaffected.

Innumerable sources of error are associated with BP measurement; see Tables 2.12–2.16.

Problems and solutions. A discussion of some of these problems and their solutions follows.

1. If the pressure on the dial refuses to rise even after eight squeezes on the bulb, the valve may have been left open. Screw it down clockwise as far as can be done comfortably.
2. If the valve is *leaky*, there will be a transient rise in dial reading after each squeeze, followed by a decline, often with some hissing as air escapes the system.

Table 2.12
Causes of Artifacts in Blood Pressure Measurement

Artifacts due to equipment
Inadequately tested or calibrated systems
Mercury/gravity or aneroid sphygmomanometer defects: clogged
  air vent; improper calibration; incompletely deflated bladder;
  faulty tubing, inflation system, or exhaust valve; insufficient mercury in reservoir; failure to "zero" indicator
Cuff size/arm size disparity: limb circumference-to-cuff width ratio
  of greater than 2.5 produces falsely high indirect pressure readings

Artifacts due to examiner technique
Unsupported arm gives falsely higher pressure
Examiner positions instrument at level above or below heart or
  presses stethoscope too firmly over vessel
Examiner has preference for even-numbered digits, etc.
Cold hands of examiner or cold equipment raises blood pressure
Subject-examiner interaction affects pressure reading
Acoustic monitoring system is impaired

3. If the cuff has been placed on backwards (inside out), the bladder will expand grotesquely when being pumped up, making a balloon-like enlargement of the cuff that will pull open the Velcro attachments.

4. Measurement over clothing produces acoustic and manometric artifacts.

5. Working around tangled instruments wastes time and promotes measurement errors.

6. Too-high inflation may cause pain and amplify the "white-coat effect" that produces a higher BP.

7. If the SBP has been estimated by palpation, you will not misconstrue the low end of an **auscultatory gap** as the SBP. Keep listening for 30 torr below the last audible Korotkoff sound. If further Korotkoff sounds appear, you have crossed an auscultatory gap, and the DBP is redefined by the (new) last audible sound.

8. In atrial fibrillation, multiple readings may be necessary.

Orthostatic Pulse and Blood Pressure Measurements

Goals. Determine the intravascular volume status and autonomic function.

Table 2.13
Common Sources of Variation in Blood Pressure Measurement

Instrument Source	Cause	Effect	Method to Rectify
Manometer	Loss of mercury	Reading impaired	Have medical equipment dealer add mercury to 0 mark
	Clogged air vent at top of manometer tube	Mercury column will respond sluggishly to pressure	Clean or replace air vent
	Loose air vent nut	Mercury column will bounce	Tighten knurled nut at top of column
Bladder	Too narrow	High reading	Determine bladder and cuff size
	Too wide	Low reading	Determine bladder and cuff size
	Not centered over artery	High reading	Use proper technique
Cuff	Loose application	High reading	Use proper technique
	Applied over clothing	Reading impaired	Use proper technique
	Too narrow	High reading	Use large adult cuff
	Too wide	Low reading	Use pediatric cuff
Tubing	Pressure leaks	Reading impaired	Check for leaks and replace
Stethoscope	Eartips not forward	Auditory impairment; low systolic, high diastolic	Use proper technique

Table 2.14
Patient Characteristics That Falsely Elevate Blood Pressure

Pain	Recent exercise	Chilling
Full bladder or rectum	Sleeplessness	Recent smoking
Auscultatory gap	Fear of health visit	Adverse interaction with health professional

Table 2.15
Patient Characteristics That Falsely Reduce Blood Pressure

Recent eating
Volume depletion
Auscultatory gap (lower end misconstrued as SBP)

Table 2.16
Contraindications to Using a Limb for Blood Pressure Measurement

Intravenous line in place	Local lymphedema
Arteriovenous fistula for hemodialysis	Local thrombophlebitis
	Recent fracture or trauma to the limb
Mastectomy or axillary dissection on this side	Brachial artery bruit

Technique. With the patient supine, count the pulse and measure the BP. If the patient is hypotensive or tachycardiac in the supine position, stop! In this setting, orthostatic checks are contraindicated and dangerous. If this is not the case, have the patient sit and dangle his legs over the side of the table or chair, then repeat the measurements. If they are unchanged, have the patient stand, then repeat the measurements.

Deconditioning. The mild exertion of sitting up or arising will transiently increase heart rate in the sedentary, in the deconditioned, and in those with cardiac problems. Purposeful delay in measurement for 1 minute after transfer minimizes false-positive results. If the patient has difficulty standing, offer a hand to hold, a cane, or a walker, or have the patient lean against an examining table for support throughout the upright part of the test.

Interpretation. Slight rise in pulse rate, a dip in SBP of 10 or less, and steady or slightly increased DBP are all normal responses to assuming the upright posture. Marked rise in pulse rate is **orthostatic tachycardia;** this has the same significance as does orthostatic hypotension. The same rise in pulse rate plus a drop in DBP and/or a drop in SBP of more than 15 torr is characteristic of intravascular **volume depletion**. *BP drops without compensatory pulse rises are characteristic of* **autonomic neuropathy.** See Table 2.17.

Table 2.17
Common Settings of Orthostatic Hypotension

Old age, particularly among hypertensive patients
Antihypertensive medication
Mineralocorticoid deficiency
Other medicines, e.g., phenothiazines, tricyclic antidepressants

Orthostatic tachycardia. With good vascular tone and reflexes, intravascular volume depletion is often compensated by maintenance of BP at the expense of increasing the heart rate. Orthostatic tachycardia can occur with or without orthostatic hypotension in hypovolemia.

Caveats. If orthostatic abnormalities are demonstrated on transferring the patient from the supine to the seated position, there is no diagnostic gain in proceeding to the standing position, and there is risk. If the test produces chest pain or a sense of impending syncope ("brownout"), the test is terminated, and the patient is returned to the supine position. Reproduction of dizziness and minor faintness do not require termination until immediately after a first postsymptom measurement. This sequence will conclusively demonstrate whether the symptom correlates with orthostatic changes or not.

If symptoms occur on arising from a chair, omit the supine measurement and proceed directly from the seated to the standing position. Orthostatic changes are sometimes demonstrable in the standing position only and, occasionally, only on maintaining that position for 3 minutes.

Orthostatic BP checks without orthostatic pulse checks are meaningless.

When autonomic dysfunction is present, it is impossible to assess for hypovolemia via orthostatic checks. See Table 2.18. If orthostatic hypotension is found, but the pulse has not been counted in both positions, the examiner cannot discriminate between hypovolemia and autonomic dysfunction.

The settings in which to suspect hypovolemia include all causes of decreased fluid intake or increased fluid output or fluid loss, the key elements of which are listed in Tables 2.19 and 2.20.

Table 2.18
Common Settings of Autonomic Dysfunction

Old age
Diabetes mellitus
Other peripheral neuropathies, especially
  B_{12} deficiency
Use of autonomic blockers such as
  atenolol or terazosin
Use of medicines with autonomic side
  effects, e.g., tricyclic antidepressants,
  neuroleptics

Table 2.19
Causes of Decreased Oral Intake

Anorexia	Lack of food	Odynophagia
Malaise	Environmental	Nausea
	water deprivation	Oral pain
	Hypodipsia	

Table 2.20
Causes of Increased Fluid Loss

Excess diuretic medication
Increased insensible loss with fever or diaphoresis
Blood donation
Vomiting
Diarrhea
Loss into an internal wound or other third-space collection
External drainage

Pulsus Paradoxus Measurement

Goals. Determine the presence of chest disease sufficient to tax cardiorespiratory function.
Technique.
1. Take the BP in the usual way.
2. Deflate the cuff completely for 30 seconds.
3. Reinflate the cuff to 20 torr above SBP.
4. Deflate the cuff slowly, listening for the very first tap of a Korotkoff sound during expiration only, expecting silence during inspiration if the cuff is then locked. This is the **expiratory SBP.**

5. Deflate the cuff 10 torr and relock.
6. Listen again.
   a. If Korotkoff sounds are still audible only in expiration, there is an abnormal pulsus paradoxus.
   b. If, however, Korotkoff sounds are heard throughout the respiratory cycle, you are clearly at or below the **inspiratory SBP,** and the difference between the inspiratory and expiratory SBPs lies within normal range; i.e., the patient does not have an abnormal pulsus paradoxus.

Interpretation. A difference of 0–8 torr between SBP in expiration (higher) and inspiration (lower) is normal. A difference of more than 10 constitutes an abnormal pulsus paradoxus. See Table 2.21 for differential diagnosis of the same.

Table 2.21
Principal Causes of Pulsus Paradoxus

Severe chronic **obstructive airway disease**, e.g., emphysema
Severe **asthma**
Heart failure of any cause, particularly when severe
Cardiomyopathy
Cardiac tamponade
Pericardial constriction (inconstant)
Shock

3

Examination of the Skin

The skin has unique features. It is highly and continuously accessible, provided we take the trouble to have the patient disrobe. It illustrates the principle, "Examine regionally, think systemically"; i.e., although many skin lesions have no systemic significance, you as examiner must think systemically.

Goals. Identify lesions of importance and distinguish them from a background of common variants and minor imperfections of no medical importance.

Technique. *Inspection.* Inspection, the chief method for this examination, requires good light, a magnifying glass, a ruler for measurement of lesions, and full exposure to light and to the eye and hand of the examiner. Fluorescent lighting is better than incandescent lighting, but both produce more false-positive and false-negative results than inspection in daylight.

Lesions are characterized as to size, shape, margins, elevation, color, body location, distribution, and other distinguishing characteristics. Along with the verbal description, a sketch is often made to enhance communication and memory.

Palpation. Palpation calls for disposable plastic gloves if there is any question of infectivity. Gloves are vital for palpation of genitalia or oral mucosa.

After palpation, a lesion is further characterized as to textural characteristics, induration, fixation to adjacent structures, and fluctuance.

A subset of palpation consists in determining whether a lump is intracutaneous or subcutaneous. If the skin can be slid over it, the mass is subcutaneous; if the skin moves with it, it is either intracutaneous or tethered to the skin.

Magnification. Magnification may reveal, for example, details of pigmentation.

Diascopy. **Diascopy** consists of pressing a flat transparent lens or other object against a lesion. It helps you as examiner to see how much of a red or purple lesion represents intravascular blood.

Wood's light. **Wood's light**, an ultraviolet light source, highlights certain features indistinguishable in ambient light. Let the light warm up, darken the room, and then attend to published precautions.

Interpretation. The enormous list of possibilities is reduced by "dividing and conquering" on the basis of sites and characteristics of lesions. Tables 3.1–3.15 employ this strategy. The mastery of some standard terminology is indispensable to allow such groupings.

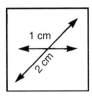

Dimensions (measured for accuracy), including height if any elevation

Configuration

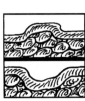

Elevation

or

Depression

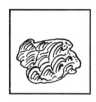

Palpable characteristics, if any, e.g., **smoothness, induration, tenderness**

Color(s)

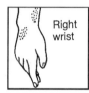

Body location(s)

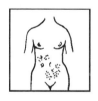

Pattern of distribution

Flat (Nonpalpable) Lesions

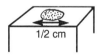

Macule: circumscribed discoloration less than 1 cm in largest dimension

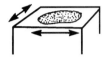

Patch: same but larger than 1 cm

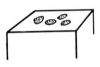

Petechiae (singular, *petechia*): purple to red spots, each less than 0.5 cm, usually occurring in groups; sometimes palpable, sometimes not

Purpura: purple to red discolorations less than 0.5 cm each (may be faintly palpable)

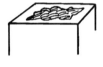

Ecchymoses (bruises): purple to red zones of discoloration under an intact epithelial surface

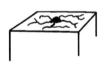

Spider angioma: red spot with radiating "legs" that blanches with central pressure and fills from the center (spot in center may be palpable)

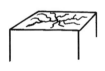

Venous "spider": superficial collection of tiny veins in stellate configuration; empties with pressure, fills slowly from the periphery

Raised Solid Lesions

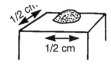

Papule: less than 1 cm in diameter

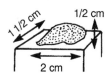

Plaque: greater than 1 cm in diameter but confined to the superficial dermis

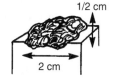

Nodule: greater than 1 cm in diameter, deeper in the dermis than a plaque and/or extending farther upward from the skin surface

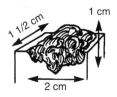

Tumor: a nodule that is poorly demarcated or about which you suspect a neoplastic origin; or larger than 2 cm in greatest dimension

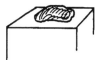

Wheal: pink to very pale, slightly elevated, circumscribed area of skin edema

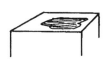

Scale: flaky heap of keratinized cells that exfoliate with scraping (can occur at surface of plaque or patch or by itself)

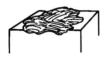

Crust: elevated dried exudate of blood, serum, or pus (usually on surface of lesion, although it may be seen on its own)

Raised Cystic Lesions

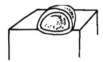

Vesicle: surface elevation filled with clear fluid, less than 1 cm in diameter

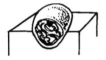

Pustule: same but filled with purulent (yellow, viscous to solid) content

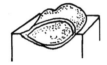

Bulla: same as vesicle but greater than 1 cm in diameter

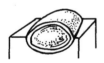

Cyst: encapsulated fluid-filled (rather than solid) mass

Depressed Lesions

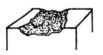

Atrophy: loss of skin markings and of skin thickness, often with a pale, shiny surface

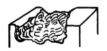

Erosion: area, often but not inevitably moist, of superficial loss of epidermis

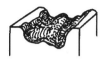 **Ulcer:** area of loss of epidermis and dermis, forming a crater of any dimension (may be depressed, flat, or elevated)

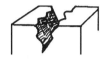 **Fissure:** narrow, linear crack in epidermis with exposure of dermis

Where on the body surface do the lesions appear; i.e., are they generalized over all parts of the body or localized to one or more of the following areas?

- Palms and/or soles (or excepting palms and soles)
- Intertriginous areas/moist skin folds
- Extensor surfaces only
- Trunk only
- Face and neck or malar area only
- Pressure areas, as where tight clothing chafes or where the weight of the bed-bound patient presses
- Skin appendages (fingernails, toenails, hair, eyebrows, and lashes)
- Mucous membranes (conjunctiva, mouth, vagina, anterior urethra, anus)

What is the distribution of the lesions? The following sketches show the various patterns of distribution.

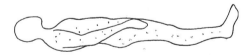

Scattered and generalized

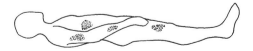

Confluent (coalescent), i.e., multiple lesion blending together

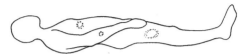

Annular, i.e., in ring formation(s)

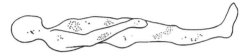

Clustered, occurring in a group or groups different from any of the prior patterns

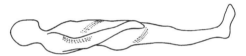

Linear, i.e., occurring in streaks

The commonest and most important lesions are listed in each table, but the categorizations are not absolute; i.e., any lesion can appear elsewhere than in the "classic" site or with a morphology other than that described here. Learning subtleties and variants takes far more time and space than is available here.

Diascopy. If a lesion consists principally of vascular congestion, it will blanch as externally applied pressure drives red cells into adjacent vessels. Failure to blanch suggests either that red cells are extravasated or that abnormal microvasculature does not permit free passage of cells.

Wood's light. Interpretations of lesions with the aid of the Wood's light are listed in Table 3.15.

Skin color. Normal skin color is often darker in intertriginous areas and on the genital, areolar, and perianal skin. Dark-skinned persons often have a bluish tinge to the lips and nailbeds. Heat, excitement, or embarrassment may flush the skin of the face and upper torso a dull to bright red, as may the vascular instability of perimenopausal "hot flashes."

Alteration in texture. Skin turgor varies with hydration and age, so that when in the elderly the skin is pinched, "tenting" may be present but may not signify extravascular fluid volume depletion.

Sun-exposed skin, unless artificially oiled, becomes drier and somewhat coarser than does protected skin. "Dry skin" often signifies roughening rather than loss of moisture.

Table 3.1
Macules and Other Flat Lesions

Name	Characteristics	Associations
"Birthmarks"	Slightly raised, usually irregular discolorations; color varies	
Café-au-lait spots	Flat, pale tan irregular patches	Neurofibromatosis if large/numerous
Chloasma	Darkening of skin around eyes and malar regions	Pregnancy, oral contraceptive
Lentigines	Brownish macules, especially on hands, arms, face	Age, solar damage
Nevus	Brown, uniform, raised or flat	Age?
Striae		
Bland ("stretch marks")	Abdomen, thighs, irregular; pale bland variety distinct from purple pigmented ones	Pregnancy, other weight gain
Purple	Abdomen; this form also produced by pregnancy or weight gain	Usually from glucocorticoid excess
Telangiectases	Dilation and twisting of superficial capillaries	Age, solar damage
Vitiligo	Patchy complete loss of melanin pigmentation	Endocrinopathies; also idiopathic

Table 3.2
Papular, Cystic, and Nodular Lesions (See Also Table 3.7 for Other
Key Entries)

Name	Characteristics	Associations
Acne	Variably open, papular, pustular, cystic	Oily skin
Cherry hemangiomas	Small, bright red papules, especially on trunk	None
Common warts	Rough frond-like surface usual except on soles	Papillomavirus
Corns and calluses	Heaped-up keratin, especially on hands and feet	Trauma, pressure
Keloid	Exuberant scar, white to dark surface, soft	Black persons
Lipomas	Soft, often feel intracutaneous	Usually none
Sebaceous cysts	Pore at exit point on skin sometimes visible; soft but not fluctuant	Rarely in polyposis syndromes
Seborrheic keratoses	Raised, rough, greasy, brown to black	Solar damage
Skin tags	Fleshy, smooth, and partially pedunculated	Age; no clear relation to colon polyps
Xanthomas	Protean, often covered by smooth epithelium, variable size/locale	Hyperlipidemia

Table 3.3
Scales, Plaques, and Erosions

Name	Characteristics	Associations
Lichenification	Thickened, hyperkeratotic	Rubbing/scratching, sometimes eczema
Psoriasis	Silvery scale alternating with erythema	
Seborrheic dermatitis	Red-yellow greasy scale, especially on eyebrows, forehead, elsewhere on head, face, chest	Usually none
Solar (senile, actinic) keratosis	Sandpapery-feeling, flat to slightly raised, roughened, brownish area	Solar damage

Table 3.4
Vesicular and Bullous Lesions and Rashes

Condition	Comments or Caveats
INFECTIOUS DISEASES	
Viral	
Herpes simplex virus	Localized, vesicular, intensely painful
Herpes genitalis	Variant of simplex occurring in perineal zone
Herpes zoster virus	
Chickenpox (varicella)	Generalized; crops of erupting vesicles, fever
Shingles	Typically dermatomal vesicles
Molluscum contagiosum	Umbilicated lesions; vesiculation is less conspicuous
Bacterial	
With erysipelas	Minor component: erythema, skin edema predominate
With impetigo (transient)	Less conspicuous than purulent ulcers
DIRECT TRAUMA	
Overlying fractures	Associated with extensive skin hemorrhage, "blood blisters"
Common blisters	Bullae, usually on feet, associated with marked exercise or trauma
Associated with barbiturate overdose	One of several patterns of injury associated with these agents and with coma
With pressure ulcers	Setting crucial
IMMUNE INJURY	
Drug hypersensitivity reactions	Many medicines may produce these
Eczematous contact dermatitis	Vesicles among erosions, scale, erythema
Dyshidrotic eczema (pompholyx)	Same, with history of frequent immersion, often on hand(s)
PRIMARY BULLOUS DISORDERS	
Dermatitis herpetiformis	Associated with celiac disease; extensor surfaces, papules and vesicles
Bullous pemphigoid	Intact large bullae usually readily found
Pemphigus vulgaris	Intact bullae rare; shaggy, ruptured or flaccid bullae are found
Epidermolysis bullosa	Usually lifetime history; many variants

Table 3.5
Nail Alterations

Name	Characteristics	Association
Beau's lines and Mees' lines	White transverse lines that are seen or felt	Any disturbance of metabolism
Clubbing	Flattening of hyponychial angle; Schamroth's sign; ballottability of nailbed	Lung cancer, cyanotic heart disease, cirrhosis, other
Half-and-half nails	Bilateral brown discoloration of distal portions of nails; can be mistaken for fecal staining or nicotine	Aging and almost any disease
Nail pits	Tiny nontraumatic indentations	Psoriasis, other skin disorders
Nicotine stains	Cigarette-holding hand only, extrinsic yellow-brown discoloration	Cigarette smoking
Onychauxis	Irregularly thickened, ridged, yellowed nail	Ischemia, infection
Onychogryphosis	Same as onychauxis, but so elongated and recurved as to resemble ram's horn	Defective personal care
Onycholysis	Fraying of distal (free) edge of nail	Hyperthyroidism
Onychomycosis	Similar to onychauxis, often toenails	Fungal infection
Paronychia	Erythema, pus at margin of nail, boggy and swollen	Ingrown toenails in some cases
Pigmented bands	Transverse bands of brown to black color, grow out with nail	Associated with some drugs, e.g., cancer chemotherapy
Red lunulae	Remainder of nail normal or half-and-half	Congestive heart failure
Subungual hematoma	Black or reddish under nailbed (with appropriate history)	Trauma
White nails	Entire nail including lunula is whitened	Cirrhosis

Table 3.6
Alterations of Hair

Name	Characteristics	Association
Falling out of clumps of head hair	Pull with only moderate force at a few hairs to validate symptom report	Scalp/skin disorders, SLE,[a] chemotherapy effect
Large escutcheon	Suspect hyperestrinism/androgen excess only if accompanied by clitoral hypertrophy, undue acne, voice and somatic changes	Normal variant; sex steroid excess
Loss of body hair	Thinning or even loss of axillary hair common; of pubic hair less common	Endocrinopathies; normal aging (variable)
Loss of foot/toe hair	Associated features, e.g., shiny smooth cool skin, positive Buerger's test	Arterial insufficiency
Male pattern baldness	Medically insignificant in men, seldom significant in women	Androgen effect
Queen Anne's sign	Loss of the lateral third of the eyebrows, not from grooming activities	Hypothyroidism

[a]SLE, **systemic lupus erythematosus.**

Table 3.7
Hemorrhagic Rashes and Lesions in Febrile Patients

Condition and Classification	Comments or Caveats
INFECTIOUS DISEASES	
Bacterial	
Meningococcemia	Petechiae may coalesce into large ecchymoses
Gonococcemia	Pustules often prominent; skin lesions may be scant
Staphylococcal bacteremia	Skin involvement variable, Janeway/Osler's nodes
Bacterial endocarditis	
Pseudomonal bacteremia	Part of **ecthyma gangrenosum**
Subbacterial, e.g., rickettsial	
Rocky Mountain spotted fever	Predilection for wrists, ankles
Typhus	Rose spots
Viral	
Enteroviremias, e.g., Coxsackie A virus	Skin involvement not classical, can have pustules, vesicles
Hemorrhagic measles	Mechanism of variant unclear
IMMUNE DISORDERS	
Systemic lupus erythematosus	Petechiae may reflect vasculitis, thrombocytopenia, or both
Drug hypersensitivity reactions	Usually hypersensitivity vasculitis
Purpura fulminans	Particularly rapid, malevolent variant, often with DIC[a]
OTHER	
Fat embolism syndrome	Petechiae; neurologic, respiratory compromise usually seen

[a]DIC, disseminated intravascular coagulation.

Table 3.8
Widespread Skin Abnormalities

Name	Characteristics	Association
Drug rashes	Often widespread pale pink macules and papules, sometimes irregular distribution	Penicillins, others
Enanthems	Similar to exanthems, but with mucous membrane involvement as well	Several viruses
Exanthems	Measles spreads innumerable tiny papules downward from hairline	Measles, others
Exfoliative erythroderma	Whole body bright red; often with associated mucous membrane problems	Multiple (drug rash, paraneoplastic, etc.)
Hemorrhagic rashes		See Table 3.7

Table 3.9
Localized Skin Problems: Head and Neck Area

Name	Characteristics	Association
Actinic (solar) keratoses	Reddish to light-brown, sandpapery rough feel, flat to slightly raised	Solar damage
Basal cell cancer	Pearly masses; telangiectases common on surfaces	Solar damage
Ephelides	Flat, tiny brown freckles	?Solar damage
Heliotrope sign	Purplish eyelids and nearby skin	Dermatomyositis
Kaposi's sarcoma	Protean: blue-purple to bright-red, may start at tip of nose, in mouth, elsewhere	HIV infection
Lentigines	Small brown freckle-like areas	?Solar damage
Lentigo maligna	Melanoma in situ: typically has "ABCD" abnormalities (see Table 3.10)	Solar damage
Malar rash	Malar erythema	Lupus, eczema, mitral disease
Malignant melanoma	ABCD criteria: see Table 3.10	Solar damage
Melanocytic nevi	Well-demarcated, usually uniform brown flat to raised lesions	?Solar
Rosacea	Acne plus telangiectases, sometimes develops into rhinophyma	Often none; sometimes alcohol abuse
Seborrheic dermatitis	Red-yellow greasy scale, especially on eyebrows, forehead, elsewhere on head, face, chest	Usually none
Seborrheic keratoses	Raised, rough, greasy brown-to-black, warty; feel "stuck on"	Solar damage
Solar elastosis	Crosshatched deep indentations on back of neck	Solar damage
Squamous cell cancer	Nodules, often ulcerated, heaped margins	Solar damage

Table 3.10
Characteristics Suspicious for Malignant Melanoma, the ABCD
Schema

Asymmetry
Borders irregular
Color is very deep brown, black, highly variegated, red-white-and-
  blue, or there are areas of depigmentation
Diameter over 6 mm in greatest dimension (size of pencil eraser)

Table 3.11
Localized Skin Problems: Breasts and Axillae

Name	Characteristics	Association
Breast cancer	Uncommonly produces ulceration, retraction, or appearance similar to mastitis	
Hidradenitis suppurativa	Inflamed, tender, purulent axillary pores	Bacterial infection
Inframammary dermatitis	Erythematous, tender, often eroded	Moisture, obesity
Mastitis	Bright red, very tender breast and nipple	Lactation
Paget's disease	Nipple and areola surfaces reddened, often superficially eroded	Breast cancer
Post-inflammatory darkening	Brown flat discoloration	Prior irritation
Prominent mammary veins	When thrombosed, constitute Mondor's disease	Normal pregnancy and lactation
Skin tags	Common in axilla	None

Table 3.12
Localized Skin Problems: Back, Perineum, Perianal and Genital Areas

Name	Characteristics	Association
Atrophic vulvitis	Yellow-white, friable discoloration, often with similar vaginal change and petechiae	Old age, estrogen deficiency
Bedsores	See Table 3.13 for Shea criteria	Immobility
Chancre	Solitary genital ulcer, typically nontender, sometimes with gray base	*Treponema pallidum* infection
Collateral arteries	Large subcutaneous arteries between shoulder blades; specific, not sensitive	Coarctation of aorta
External hemorrhoids	Gray-blue to flesh-colored papules near the anal verge, sometimes ulcerated, sometimes thrombosed	Straining at stool
Fissure in ano	Exquisitely tender minute linear break	None
Fistula in ano	Ragged, inflamed defect in the perianal area	Crohn's disease
Fordyce spots	Tiny red scrotal cherry hemangiomas	None in adults
Genital herpes	Painful, tender vesicles on erythematous base	Herpes simplex virus infection
Genital warts	Warty pink masses, small, sometimes flat	Human papilloma-virus infection
Pilonidal cysts	Prominent fold of skin and tissue with central pore, sometimes discharging	None
Vulvar dystrophies	White to pink to gray flat focal discolorations	Some human papillomavirus infection, others not

Table 3.13
Shea Classification of Pressure Ulcers (Bedsores)

Grade	Characteristics
1	Nonblanchable erythema, characteristically in pressure area
2	Frank ulceration, confined to the skin
3	Ulceration extending into subcutaneous fat
4	Ulceration extending to muscle, bone, or viscus

Table 3.14
Localized Skin Problems: Legs and Feet

Name	Characteristics	Association
Cellulitis	Erythema, heat, tenderness, loss of skin markings, often with swelling	Bacterial infection
Dermatitis venosa	Numerous tiny to confluent rust-colored macules on shin, often with thickened irregular surface	Chronic venous insufficiency
Diabetic foot ulcers	Most often on soles, often over metatarsal heads; variably purulent and fibrinous	Diabetes mellitus
Erythema nodosum	Nodules deep in subcutaneous fat of shins, mild overlying erythema or brown discoloration	Multiple: sarcoid, vasculitides, tuberculosis, etc.
Gangrene	Blackening and dulling of surface	Ischemia
Shin spots	Sunken pale brown ovoid atrophic zones, on shins	Diabetes mellitus
Tinea pedis (athlete's foot)	Maceration, cracking especially between toes, desquamation of white epithelium	Superficial fungal infection
Venous ulcers	Shallow to deep epithelial defects, sometimes with heaped margins	Chronic venous insufficiency

Table 3.15
Wood's Light Findings[a–c]

Process	Color Under Wood's Light
Vitiligo	Bright white, sometimes with blue tinge
Postinflammatory hyperpigmentation	Purplish brown
Pseudomonas infection	Blue-green to blue
Erythrasma	Coral pink-red
Tinea versicolor	Yellow to golden-orange

[a]False-negative errors can result from washing within the previous 24 hours. Inadequate darkening of the room can also produce false-negatives, as can holding the light source more than 10 cm from the area to be checked.
[b]Topical products can create false-positives.
[c]The light should not be shined on the cornea.

4

Head, Eyes, Ears, Nose, Oral Cavity, and Throat (HEENT)

HEAD AND SCALP

Goals. Determine the contour, size, and shape of the cranium, the amount and distribution of the hair, and the health of the scalp.

Technique. Palpate the patient's cranium; palpate the hair and tug a few strands gently. In older persons, palpate the temporal arteries anterior to the tragus.

Interpretation.
- Common variants
  Minor side-to-side asymmetry
- Abnormalities
  Developmental abnormalities
  Frontal bossing, unusual prominence or curvature of
      forehead
    May be normal variant
    Seen in sickle cell anemia
    Seen as part of HIV embryopathy complex
  Upper head disproportionately large
    Hydrocephalus
    Paget's disease of bone
  Subcutaneous masses
    Epidermal inclusion cysts (sebaceous cysts)
    Lipomas
    Gardner's syndrome

FACE

Goals. Determine symmetry at rest and with movement; inspect for skin lesions.

Technique. Inspect the frontal and lateral aspects of the patient's face; use a magnifying glass if needed.

Interpretation.

* Common variants

    Minor side-to-side asymmetry, static

* Abnormalities of symmetry

    Side-to-side asymmetry, static and with movement (see Cranial Nerve VII)

    Nasal deviation, usually from old fracture

    Prognathia

    Macrognathia

    Micrognathia

    Swelling and crepitus *without* erythema

    Communication between air-containing sinus and subcutis

    Ethmoid sinus fracture (beneath eye)

    Swelling and crepitus *with* erythema

    Cellulitis

    Visible or palpable parotid enlargement

    Starvation, including anorexia nervosa and bulimia

    Sjögren's syndrome

    Alcoholism

    Diabetes mellitus

    Acute parotitis

    HIV infection

    Striking facial dysmorphism

    Fetal alcohol syndrome (with hypoplasia of philtrum, hypertelorism)

    Acromegaly (hypertrophic jaw, overhanging forehead and brows, coarse features)

    Hypothyroidism (puffy, apathetic facies, coarse dry skin, loss of lateral third of brows)

    Loss of lateral third of brows (Queen Anne's sign)

    Normal variant

    Hypothyroidism

    Eyebrow plucking

    Leprosy (rare)

    Severe facial edema

    Allergy

Angioedema
Anasarca of any cause
Myxedema
Superior vena caval obstruction
Morbid obesity may simulate edema

EYES AND PERIORBITAL STRUCTURES

Goal. Determine symmetry, normality, and function of the patient's eyes and periorbital structures.
Technique. Inspect the structures; palpate the orbits.
Interpretation.
- Normal variants
  Globe: range of normal protrusion
  Sclera, cornea, iris
    Pinguecula
    Arcus cornealis in persons over age 50
    Iridodonesis secondary to cataract surgery
  Pupils
    Congenital anisocoria with normal direct and consensual normal light reactions
- Abnormalities
    Eyelids
      Hordeolum
      Ectropion
      Ptosis
    Conjunctiva
    Chemosis (edema)
      Allergic
      Local irritation
      Superior vena caval syndrome
      Respiratory failure
    Irritation
    Bacterial or viral infection
    Physical irritation
    Chemical or particulate; Sjögren's
    Exophthalmos, symmetric
    Graves' hyperthyroidism
    Congestive heart failure
    Exophthalmos, unilateral or asymmetric

Graves' hyperthyroidism
Ocular neoplasm
Inflammatory lesions
Orbital pseudotumor

Inspection of the Superior Conjunctiva

Goal. Enlarge area of visible conjunctiva.

Technique. Have the patient look away. Place a cotton swab firmly against the patient's lid, grasp the patient's lashes, and fold that section of the patient's lid over the swab-stick.

"Nipple Test"

Goal. Demonstrate shallow anterior chamber for planned pupillodilation, to avoid precipitating acute angle-closure glaucoma.

Technique. Shine a light medially across the globe at the level of limbus. Observe for casting of the medial iris into shadow (Fig. 4.1).

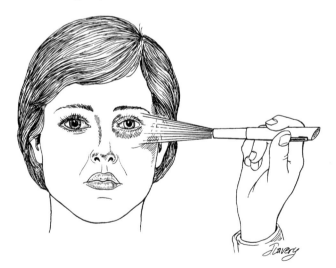

Figure 4.1 "Nipple" test to determine depth of anterior chamber.

Interpretation. The presence of shadowing indicates that the iris is standing forward from the surface of the globe; thus the anterior chamber is shallow, and pupillodilation by the generalist is contraindicated.

Funduscopic Examination

Goal. Inspect anterior chamber, lens, retina and vessels, optic nerve head, and macula.

Technique.

1. Have the patient seated at approximately your eye level, with room lights dimmed. Instruct the patient to focus on a designated distant point.
2. Cast the light beam from the side, to inspect anterior chamber.
3. Hold the ophthalmoscope in your right hand, and using your right eye, inspect the patient's right eye. When finished, change hands and eyes and examine the patient's left eye.
4. Hold the instrument 30 cm from the patient, with diopter indicator at +10. Move the light gradually toward the patient, seeking the red reflex.
5. Adjust the diopters down as the fundus comes into view.
6. Study the fundus systematically by quadrants for
   a. *Veins and arteries:* Size, crossings, irregularities, and venous pulsations
   b. *Retina:* Color, uniformity of pigmentation, discolorations, lesions
   c. *Optic disc:* Smoothness of margins, colors, and focus relative to surrounding retina

Interpretation. Lens. The lens should be transparent, thus invisible. Lenticular opacities (cataracts) form black holes in the red reflex.

Veins and arteries. Venous pulsations are seen in many normal persons. Absence of pulsations may also be normal but in the proper setting raises the question of increased intracranial pressure. Tortuosity may be seen with hyperviscosity states, in sickle cell disease, and as a normal variant.

Retina. The darkness of the retina parallels skin melanin.
- *Hemorrhages*

    Small dot hemorrhages are seen in many disorders, such as severe hypertension, diabetes mellitus, leukemia, and severe anemia.

    Flame-shaped hemorrhages are most commonly seen in severe hypertension.

    Hemorrhages with a white center ("Roth spots") occur in infective endocarditis, leukemia, severe anemia, and scurvy.

- *Exudates*

    Soft, "cotton-wool spots" are flat and white, have indistinct edges, and obscure the subjacent retina and vessels. They are seen in microvasculopathies such as diabetes, hypertension, renal disease, vasculitis, and the severe anemia of AIDS.

    Hard "exudates" have sharp edges and are more yellowish than soft exudates, may be shiny, and vary in size. They are seen with leaky microvessels, microvasculopathies, many infectious diseases, and some primary eye diseases.

Pupillodilation

Goal. Enhance inspection of the retina.

Technique. If you are planning to perform pupillodilation, ask whether the patient has had cataract surgery and a lens implant. If so, **do not dilate the pupil.**

1. Pick a time at which the patient will be available a half hour later.

2. Ask the patient about any history of acute angle-closure glaucoma. If the response is positive, consult an ophthalmologist before proceeding. A successful dilation within the past 2 years strongly suggests that the patient will tolerate the procedure well.

3. Infer the anterior chamber depth by the nipple test (see above). A positive nipple test means dilation is risky and should be done, if at all, by an ophthalmologist. Pupil size and the direct and consensual

pupillary light reactions of each eye are recorded as baseline measurements.

4. Warn the patient that the drops sometimes sting briefly but that this will abate and that vision will be impaired, with some photophobia, for an hour or two after the examination. Inform the patient, family, and nurse that this test may rarely unmask acute angle-closure glaucoma. Failure of vision to improve, new headache, or eye pain should prompt considering this rare but important complication.

5. Have the patient lie down flat or at a 30° angle, with eyes rolled upward. Hold the solution bottle a few centimeters above the eye and instill a single drop of tropicamide 1% ophthalmic solution at the medial canthus. Have the patient blink 5 times and then keep the eye closed. If the dropper touches the patient's lash or any part of the patient's body, the bottle is bacterially contaminated and must be discarded.

6. After 25 minutes, note pupil size. Direct and consensual light reactions should have been ablated.

Note: Function of the pupil is discussed under Cranial Nerves I–XII.

EARS

Goal. Assess the external ears, canals, and tympanic membranes. Hearing and vestibular function are discussed under Cranial Nerves I–XII.

Technique. *External ear (Fig. 4.2).* Inspect and palpate the external ear.

Otoscopic examination. To perform an otoscopic examination in adults, follow these steps:

1. Place a disposable or a clean reusable speculum on the otoscope.

2. With the patient's head tipped away from you, grasp the helix of the patient's auricle and tug posterosuperiorly.

3. Introduce the speculum into the patient's ear canal under direct visualization. As the canal is traversed,

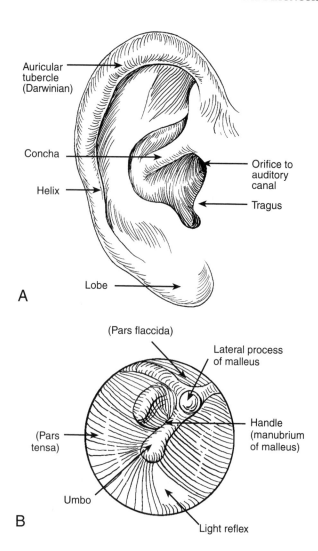

Figure 4.2 **A.** Anatomy of external ear. **B.** Otoscopic view of right tympanic membrane.

observe for scaling, erythema, bleeding points, or discharge.
4. Continue insertion of the speculum under direct visualization until the tympanic membrane is in full view.
5. Inspect the membrane for color, translucency, presence of light reflex, rupture, erythema, and bulging.

Interpretation.
- External ear abnormalities
  Lumps
    Gouty tophi of pinnae
    Benign fibromas
    Preauricular lymph node enlargement
      Otitis externa
      Adenoviral conjunctivitis
      As part of generalized lymphadenopathy
  Tender, nodular, or nonpulsatile temporal artery
    Consider giant cell arteritis
- External auditory canal
    Otitis externa: tenderness to traction, erythema, with or without exudate
    Malignant otitis externa with deep canal ulcers, exposed cartilage, sloughing
- Tympanic membrane
    Otitis media
      Light reflex and shiny surface missing
      Membrane reddened, prominent vasculature at margins
      Drum full to bulging; landmarks obscured
      Drum may be perforated; pus may be draining through perforation
    Serous otitis media
      Thin, yellow fluid visible through uninflamed membrane
    Bullous myringitis
      Blebs on surface of membrane and adjacent canal, seen in viral or other infections

Cerumen Removal

Goal. Permits accurate visual assessment of the auditory canal and tympanic membrane, to enhance hearing acuity.

Technique.

1. Instill a few drops of a ceruminolytic, e.g., a 10% solution of sodium bicarbonate in glycerol, into the affected canal.
2. Leave the patient's head tilted away from the treated ear for a few minutes and/or insert a cotton pledget to keep the agent in the canal.
3. One day later, reexamine the canal for drainage of the liquefied cerumen.
4. Gentle irrigation with warm water may be used to complete cleansing of extremely stubborn plugs. If this is unsuccessful, refer the patient to an otologist.

NOSE AND PARANASAL SINUSES

Goal. Assess nasal mucosa, septum, walls, turbinates, and sinuses.

Technique.

1. Have the patient sniff through each naris while compressing the other (demonstrates functional patency).
2. With the patient's head tilted back, press the tip of the nose to spread the nares for inspection.
3. Shine a light into each naris and inspect
     Mucosa for color, discharge, bleeding
     Septum for centrality, integrity, mucosal appearance
     Lateral walls for turbinates, meatal discharge

Interpretation.

* Blocked air passages
     Mucosal inflammation or heavy discharge
     Septal deviation
     Polyps
* Abnormal mucosal appearance
     Allergic rhinitis: pale, boggy, and grayish to mauve
     Common cold: reddening, heavy yellow-green mucoid but not purulent discharge

Rhinitis medicamentosa: red and swollen or dry and
rubbery
Acute sinusitis: pus in nose

Percussion and Transillumination of Sinuses

Goal. Assess for inflammation when the patient complains of facial pain and tenderness, frontal headache, or
unrelenting upper respiratory infection.

Technique.
* *Frontal:* Strike the tip of the flexed middle finger against
  the midpoint of the cutaneous projection of the sinus.
* *Maxillary:* Percuss each malar eminence.

  For *transilluminating the maxillary sinus*, use a completely darkened room and a penlight or a more narrow and
  directed sinus transilluminator. Place the tip of the transilluminator just under each of the patient's inferior orbital rims
  (Fig. 4.3) and look for differential transillumination of each
  antrum. Alternatively, place the tip, covered by a disposable
  glove to stay sanitary, to each side of the palate. Each time,
  the patient needs to have lips closed around the instrument
  so that transillumination can be compared from side to side.

  The *frontal sinus* is studied with a variant of the first
  method, whereby the light source is placed under the superior orbital rim.

Interpretation. Tenderness to percussion, especially if
unilateral, suggests inflammation of the sinus cavity, usually infective. Failure to transilluminate implies a thickened,
inflamed sinus lining and/or fluid and pus in the cavity.

ORAL CAVITY

Goal. Assess the lips, tongue, palate, gingivae, teeth,
and buccal mucosa.

Technique. Inspect the following in order:
* Lips
* Dorsal surface of the tongue
* Floor of the mouth
* Lateral surface of the tongue: grasp the tongue with a
  gauze pad, pull it to one side and then the other to
  view each side for color, lesions, and bleeding

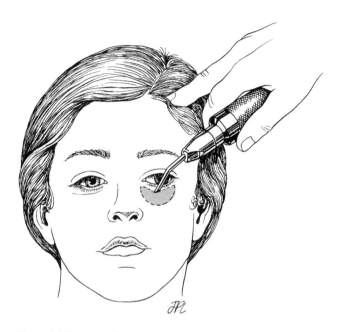

Figure 4.3 Sinus transilluminator held to inferior orbit to assess maxillary sinus.

- Palate
- Gingival surfaces and buccal mucosa
- Teeth
  Palpate the oral cavity, using the following steps:
  1. Glove both hands.
  2. With two fingers of one hand in the floor of the mouth and with the fingers of the other hand pressing cephalad from under the chin, palpate the floor of the mouth for masses, irregularities, or tenderness.
  Interpretation.
- Lips
    Angular cheilosis or cracks at the corners of the lips
      Dental malocclusion

Maceration from persistent moisture
  (drooling, etc.)
Riboflavin deficiency
Candidal infection
Carcinoma

- Tongue
  Glossitis
    Atrophic, with shiny red surface, "beefy tongue"
      of Nutritional deficiency, especially B_{12}, B_1
    Migratory atrophic ("geographic") as normal
      variant
    Inflammatory: "strawberry tongue" in scarlet
      fever, variants in other infectious diseases
- Mucosa and gingivae
  Periodontitis—boggy, erythematous, tender or puru-
    lent gingiva
  Pyorrhea—frank pus around exposed carious roots
    of teeth
  Infections
    Candidal stomatitis—white, curdy pseudomem-
      brane on surfaces that causes bleeding when
      scraped off
    Candida, atrophic—flat, red lesion under dentures
    Intraoral herpes—tiny vesicles on erythematous
      bases that, when scraped, open up to leave
      ragged shallow and painful ulcers
    Aphthous stomatitis—flat discoloration without
      vesicle, which ulcerates
    White plaque that comes off with tongue blade
      scraping, leaving normal mucosa beneath—
      food or mild staining
    White plaque that does not budge with scraping—
      consider hairy leukoplakia
    Oral cancers: may present as flat white plaques, a
      red lesion, ulceration, induration, or exophytic
      mass
  Intraoral Kaposi's sarcoma: red to red-blue to purple
    intraoral nodules; less commonly, macules; patch-
    es; in patients with known HIV disease

Oral signs of systemic disease
>   Crohn's disease: oral mucosa may become fissured
>   and cobblestoned looking; angular cheilitis;
>   persistent and severe oral aphthae
>   Bulimia and anorexia nervosa: erosions of lingual
>   surface of teeth, "etching" around fillings

AIDS
>   Pseudomembranous candidiasis very common
>   but not specific
>   Hairy leukoplakia—whitish gray roughening
>   on lateral surfaces of tongue

OROPHARYNX

Technique. The patient's mouth should be fully open.
With penlight, inspect the patient's tonsils, peritonsillar tissue, and posterior pharynx. If the dorsum of the tongue
obscures the view, ask the patient to "pant like a puppy."
Observe the color of the mucosa, size of the palatine tonsils,
or presence of any postnasal drainage, mass, erythema, or
exudate.

Interpretation.
- Infections
>   Erythema without exudate, especially with hypertro-
>   phy of posterior pharyngeal lymphoid tissue, is
>   likely to be viral; with exudate, consider bacterial
>   source more, but the clinical appearance does not
>   reliably distinguish between the two
>   Erythema with pseudomembrane formation: consider
>   diphtheria, mononucleosis
>   Erythema with a history of oral-genital sex: consider
>   gonorrheal pharyngitis
- Multiple palatal telangiectases
>   Consider cirrhosis or hereditary telangiectasia

CRANIAL NERVES I–XII

Although examination of the cranial nerves (CNs) is integrated into the head, eyes, ears, nose, and throat (HEENT)
examination sequence, systematic examination of these
nerves is presented here as a unit. See Table 4.1.

Cranial Nerve I: Olfactory

Technique. Place tobacco or ground coffee in a small bottle. Occlude one of the patient's nostrils and ask the patient to sniff the stimulus in the bottle and identify it. Repeat procedure with the other nostril.

Table 4.1
Cranial Nerves[a]

"On Old Olympus' Towering Top A Finn and German Viewed Some Hops." *Old Clinician's Mnemonic*

CN I ("On")—**Olfactory:** sense of smell
    TESTS
        See subsection Cranial Nerve I: Olfactory
CN II ("Old")—**Optic:** visual acuity
    TESTS
        Snellen chart for distance vision
        Printed card for near vision
        Visual fields (by confrontation technique)
        Component of direct and consensual pupillary light reation
CN III ("Olympus")—**Oculomotor**: motor nerve to five extrinsic eye muscles: superior rectus, inferior rectus, medial rectus, inferior oblique, and palpebrae superioris; the outermost fibers of the third cranial nerve innervate pupillary construction.
    TESTS
        Extraocular eye movements, excluding conjugate motion
        Pupillary response to light (direct and consensual) and accommodation
CN IV ("Towering")— **Trochlear:** motor nerve to superior oblique extrinsic eye muscle (downward and inward movement of eye)
    TESTS
        Extraocular eye movement
CN V ("Top")—**Trigeminal**
    TESTS
    A. Sensory to skin of face and cornea
        All sensation for facial skin representing three divisions of nerve (V1, V2, V3)
        Corneal reflex component
    B. Motor to muscules of mastication
        Bite and bulk of masseter muscle
CN VI ("A")—**Abducens:** motor to the lateral rectus muscles of eyes (lateral movement)
    TESTS
        Lateral (abducent) extraocular movement of each eye

Table 4.1 *(continued)*
Cranial Nerves[a]

CN VII ("Finn")—**Facial**
    TESTS
    A. Motor to muscles of face
        Smile—symmetry of lower facial muscle movement
        Frown—symmetry of forehead movement, tight eyelid closure
    B. Sensory for taste, anterior two-thirds of tongue
        See subsection Cranial Nerve VII: Facial
CN VIII ("And")—**Acoustic:** sensory
    TESTS
    A. Cochlear branch: hearing acuity
        Watch ticking, finger rubbing, measured audible distance
           of whisper for symmetry
    B. Vestibular branch: balance
        Nystagmus on lateral gaze (Romberg test, visible tremor,
           past pointing, abnormal results on "cerebellar" test)
CN IX ("German")—**Glossopharyngeal**
    TESTS
    A. Motor (elevation) of posterior pharynx; laryngeal musculature
        Gag reflex, deglutition, invoice quality, water swallowing
    B. Sensory: taste to posterior one-third of tongue
        See subsection Cranial Nerves IX and X:
           Glossopharyngeal and Vagus
CN X ("Viewed")—**Vagus**
    TESTS
    A. Motor: deglutition, elevation of palate, laryngeal musculature
        Say "haaat"—symmetrical elevation of palate; voice quality;
           water swallowing
    B. Sensory: pharynx and larynx
        "Gag" reflex—afferent loop
CN XI ("Some")—**Spinal accessory:** motor to trapezius and
sternomastoid muscles
    TESTS
        Rotating the head against force
        Shrugging the shoulder against force
CN XII ("Hops")—Hypoglossal: motor to the tongue
    TESTS
        Protruding the tongue in the midline
        Protruding the tongue into each cheek

---

[a]CN, Cranial nerve.

    Interpretation.
- Transient olfactory impairment
    Seen in viral or allergic rhinitis
- Persistent bilateral impairment

Normal aging
Parkinson's disease
Kallmann's syndrome
- Persistent unilateral impairment
    Local abnormality such as naris occlusion
    Frontal lobe neoplasm
    Subdural hematoma

Cranial Nerve II: Optic

Goals. Assess visual acuity; examine for integrity of peripheral vision, optic nerve and chiasm, calcarine radiation, occipital lobe function, and the afferent loop of the pupillary reflex (see Cranial Nerve III)

Technique. *Vision testing.* Test vision using the standard pocket card or "Snellen chart."

Visual fields by confrontation. Test the visual fields as follows:
1. Position yourself face to face with the patient, at eye level, 1 meter apart.
2. Have the patient cover one eye, and you cover your own mirror-image eye. Instruct the patient to look right at your open eye in order to conduct the test of peripheral vision only.
3. In this position, systematically place your free hand equidistant from the opposing faces and sequentially at the lateral (temporal), inferior, superior, and medial (nasal) extremities of arm reach. Moving your fingers or carrying an object such as pen or colored card in your hand, move your hand toward center, asking the patient to indicate when the hand or object is first seen. Initial entry into the visual field defines the boundary of the periphery being tested. Your field of vision is the control, and any discrepancy between your limits and those of the patient is noted.
4. Normal peripheral fields approximate 90° temporally, 50° nasally, 50° superiorly, and 70° inferiorly. Marked deviation or constriction compared with the

normal control (you) indicates the need for further evaluation by perimetry.

Interpretation. *Visual field cuts.* Test visual field cuts in successively more posterior order:

1. Transection of one optic nerve anterior to the chiasm produces unilateral blindness and no visual field cut contralaterally. In this sense the impact on vision is identical with disease of one globe.

2. Damage at the chiasm, classically from expansion of a pituitary mass, damages fibers from both sides just as they cross. These fibers represent the temporal half of each eye's visual field. The result is bitemporal hemianopsia.

3. Damage to the optic tract posterior to the chiasm destroys (a) fibers that have decussated from the temporal half of the contralateral eye's visual field and (b) fibers that have not decussated from the nasal half of the ipsilateral eye's visual field. The result is a **homonymous hemianopsia.** A right calcarine lesion produces loss of the left (i.e., medial, nasal) half of the field of vision for the ipsilateral right eye and loss of the left (i.e., temporal, lateral, decussating) half of the visual field of the contralateral left eye. If only a portion of the craniocaudal dimension of an optic nerve is destroyed, there will be a corresponding diminution of the loss of visual field. By this mechanism there develop **quadrantanopsic** deficits.

Cranial Nerve III: Oculomotor

Goal. Determine the integrity of the afferent (CN II) and efferent (CN III) limbs of pupillary constriction (Fig. 4.4). (The CN III contribution to extraocular muscle movement is assessed in conjunction with CNs IV and VI below.)

Technique. *Light pupillary reflex.*

1. Dim the lights in the room so that pupils dilate slightly.

2. Tell the patient to fixate on the far wall (to avoid inadvertent accommodation).

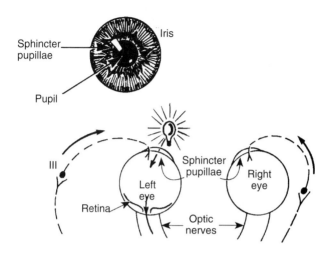

Figure 4.4 Pathways for pupillary response to light (CNs II and III).

3. A bright light source is shone directly into the right pupil. This pupil is observed for prompt and symmetrical constriction (direct pupillary response).
4. The light source is removed such that the pupil dilates again.
5. The light is shone again into the right pupil, and the left pupil is observed for prompt and symmetrical constriction (consensual pupillary response).
6. The same procedures are repeated on the other eye, illuminating the left pupil and observing both direct (left) and consensual (right) pupillary responses.

Accommodation.

1. Ask the patient to focus on the your finger held 30 cm from the patient's nose, then to follow your finger as it moves toward your nose.
2. The two pupils are observed for progressive and symmetrical constriction as the focal point moves closer to the eyes.

Interpretation. *Light reflex.* The patient with normal sight sensitivity and with an intact third nerve branch to the pupil and normal pupilloconstrictor musculature demonstrates the following normal responses:

- *Direct light response:* The pupil into which the light is shown contracts quickly to the stimulus.
- *Consensual light response:* The opposite pupil (not directly light-stimulated, only neurally stimulated) also simultaneously contracts equally.

If one eye is blind to light, it will not respond directly but should respond consensually as long as its partner's vision and its own pupilloconstrictor innervation are intact. If both eyes are blind to light, no pupillary response will occur on direct stimulus or consensually.

Asymmetry or absence of pupillary response, unless clearly accounted for on the basis of established blindness to light, indicates local or central pathology.

Accommodation. As the focal distance shortens, i.e., the object on which the eyes are focused moves closer to the eye, the pupils symmetrically and progressively contract. Failure of both or either to respond in this predictable manner is an indication for further evaluation. Blindness in either eye or in both eyes will affect this response.

Sympathetic action dilates the pupils, while parasympathetic (cholinergic) impulses constrict them. Endogenous discharge also plays a role, so that excitement with epinephrine release enlarges the pupil. Heroin produces pinpoint pupils that enlarge on administration of the opiate antagonist, naloxone. Cocaine can dilate the pupils.

Topical application of autonomic drugs to the eye affects pupil size. Ocular pilocarpine used for glaucoma constricts the pupil, as does ophthalmic timolol.

ANISOCORIA

Goal. Many persons have *physiologic anisocoria*, wherein the "resting" size of the two pupils differs enough to be recognizable on examination. There are two approaches to confirming this innocuous state: the history and the examination.

Technique. *History.* Ask if the patient or any family member has noted unequal pupils. If doubt exists, look at unretouched portrait photographs of the patient. If you discern the inequality dating from 2 or more years ago, no ominous cause is sought.

Examination. Check each pupil to see if it

1. Constricts normally in response to direct stimulation
2. Constricts consensually on illuminating the opposite eye
3. Dilates a bit after removal of the light source
4. Constricts and converges with testing of accommodation

Interpretation. If an unequal pupil does all the above, the condition is almost certainly benign anisocoria.

To determine whether it is the smaller or the larger pupil that is abnormal, a very large pupil (over 6 mm across), unless the result of topical medication, is likely to be the abnormal one. Also check extraocular motions, looking for evidence of dysfunction of the nearby cranial nerves or their effectors. Seek alterations in mental status, including change in level of consciousness, and focal neurologic deficits. Some possible underlying conditions are increased intracranial pressure, local compression by cerebral aneurysm, and neoplasia.

If accommodation (constriction on near gaze) is preserved in a large pupil whose light reaction is sluggish or absent, either **Argyll Robertson pupil** or **Adie's syndrome** is present. Neurosyphilis involving the midbrain is the most discussed cause of the Argyll Robertson pupil, although **diabetic neuropathy** is commonest. Adie's syndrome is an innocent polyneuropathy whose only other manifestations are reduced or absent knee and ankle jerks.

Marcus Gunn Pupil

Marcus Gunn pupil is a relative (i.e., incomplete) afferent pupillary defect. The leading etiology is multiple sclerosis. The ability to fire neural impulses in response to retinal illumination is reduced, often unilaterally or asymmetrically, but efferent pupilloconstriction is not. Thus, illuminating the opposite eye will cause prompt physiologic consensual pupilloconstriction of the diseased eye. Shining the light into the diseased eye, however, produces delayed or incomplete direct pupilloconstriction. If the light is moved from the unaffected eye to the abnormal eye, the pupil appears to dilate on illumination. What has really happened is that the consensual impulse to constriction from the intact pathway has been removed and nothing equally potent has replaced it.

Cranial Nerves IV and VI (Tested With III): Trochlear and Abducens

Technique. Symmetrical tracking of the eyes that permits focused binocular vision is controlled by a well-matched and integrated set of muscles regulated by three cranial nerves. Functional testing of these muscles and nerves is accomplished through the following steps:

1. Face the patient directly, at eye level, 30 cm away.
2. Using a finger or other object as the focal point, ask the patient to follow movement of the object with the eyes without moving the head.
3. Move the object systematically through six directions of motion while noting any asymmetry of eye movement. Any unilateral deviation of eyeball motion or patient complaint of double vision is recorded.

If there is an apparent deficit, repeat the test with the "normal" eye covered and see if the "abnormal" one normalizes.

Interpretation (Fig. 4.5, A and B).

FURTHER PURSUIT OF APPARENT DEFICIT

Goal. Determine the anatomic location of the apparent deficit.

Technique. Repeat extraocular testing with the normal eye covered.

Interpretation.

1. If a previously abnormal eye shows full range of motion, the problem is in the median longitudinal fasciculus of the brainstem, where conjugate movement is determined.

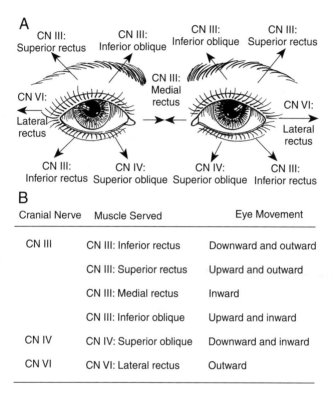

Figure 4.5 **A.** Muscles controlling eye movements. **B.** Tabular summary of nerves controlling eye movements.

2. If the deficit persists with monocular testing, consider
   CN VI or the lateral rectus muscle if there is loss of lateral gaze
   CN IV or the superior oblique muscle if there is loss of downward-inward gaze
   CN III or any of the four extraocular muscles that it innervates (inferior oblique, medial rectus, superior rectus, and inferior rectus) for any other deviation

Cranial Nerve V: Trigeminal

Goal. Assess sensory perception on the skin of the face and the function of muscles of mastication.

Technique. Sensory to the skin of the face. Test sensory perception to light touch and pain on the skin of the face.

1. *Light touch:* Pick up a cotton swab and tug out a few strands to make a fluff. Have the patient close his eyes. Instruct the patient that you will be touching him on various portions of the face. He is to indicate when he feels the cotton fluff and where he perceives the contact. Figure 4.6 indicates the three divisions of CN V on each side of the face that would be checked. Touch each skin area on each side, in random fashion, asking the patient to respond as above.

2. *Pain:* An alternative to light touch perception is that of pain in the three divisions of CN V. Using a broken swab-stick—not a pin or needle—and a firm cotton swab, ask the patient to discriminate between *sharp* and *dull.* Instructions to the patient include closure of the eyes to avoid visual cuing and a response that includes the sensation perceived— sharp or dull—and the area where the stimulus is felt, e.g., "right cheek" or "left forehead."

Motor to muscles of mastication. The masseter muscles are palpated bilaterally simultaneously as the patient bites down hard. Upon clenching the jaws, both masseter muscles become equally firm and bulky.

Corneal sensitivity. The eye normally responds to noxious stimulation of the cornea by a protective blink. This response requires intact sensory fibers of CN V and motor fibers of CN VII to the orbicularis oculi muscles. To test,

1. Pull out one fine cotton wisp from the tip of a swab.
2. Ask the patient to focus on a spot past your shoulder.
3. From the side, so it will not enter the patient's field of vision, touch the swab lightly to the patient's cornea. The eyes should blink reflexly. Test each cornea separately.

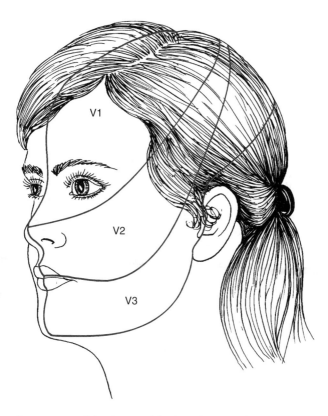

Figure 4.6 Facial distribution of the three divisions of CN V. *V1*, ophthalmic; *V2*, maxillary; and *V3*, mandibular.

Interpretation. The nuclei of CN V are set in the tight-packed pons, so that isolated fifth nerve problems without ocular palsies are likely to reflect disease of the peripheral (extra-axial) course of the nerve. The commonest problem is *dermatomal herpes*. In this condition, one or more divisions—the ophthalmic (V1), maxillary (V2), and mandibular (V3)—are affected, usually unilaterally. The lesions may not appear for the first couple of days of pain. They begin as clustered vesicles on erythematous bases, then rupture, sometimes pass through a pustular phase, crust, and dry. Ocular (corneal) involvement is a sight-threatening complication of herpes zoster in CN VI. The development of conjunctivitis, dulling of the corneal light reflex, or a corneal ulcer in the setting of facial herpes infection calls for prompt ophthalmologic consultation.

Cranial Nerve VII: Facial

Technique. Each seventh cranial nerve innervates ipsilateral muscles of the forehead, eyelid, cheek, and perioral area. To test,

    1A. Ask the patient to frown or wrinkle the brow.
         or
    1B. Ask the patient to close both eyelids and resist your attempt to lift them open. In either instance, observe for side-to-side symmetry of motion.
     2. Ask the patient to smile. Observe for symmetrical elevation of the corners of the mouth.

Interpretation. Asymmetry of the mouth, nasolabial folds, and palpebral fissure suggests facial nerve palsy on the "flattened" or less mobile side. Is it peripheral or central?

* Peripheral CN VII palsy
    Findings: Forehead involved
    Seen in: Bell's palsy, idiopathic (very common)
           Lyme disease
           Sarcoidosis
           Diabetic cranial neuropathy
           Acoustic neuroma (rare)
* Central CN VII palsy
    Findings: Only lower face involved, forehead spared
    Seen in: Cortical disease, problems with upper motor neuron (internal capsule, etc.)

Cranial Nerve VIII: Acoustic

Goal. Assess for hearing loss and vestibular dysfunction.
Technique. The screening examination for hearing loss consists of the following steps:

     1. Ask the patient to close his eyes and indicate when he first hears sound.

2. Rub your thumb and index finger together successively at 2.5-cm intervals, beginning 10 cm from the
   external ear on each side.
3. Note symmetry of acuity.

If the screening examination is abnormal, continue with
the extended examination:

1. Administer the Hearing Handicap Inventory for the
   Elderly (Table 4.2).
2. Proceed to the Rinne and Weber tests (see below).

Use the following to screen for vestibular function:

Table 4.2
Hearing Handicap Inventory for the Elderly—Screening Version

PLEASE CIRCLE THE BEST ANSWER FOR EACH QUESTION

1. Does a hearing problem cause you to feel embarrassed when
   you meet new people?
   NO   SOMETIMES   YES
2. Does a hearing problem cause you to feel frustrated when talking
   to members of your family?
   NO   SOMETIMES   YES
3. Do you have difficulty hearing when someone speaks in a whisper?
   NO   SOMETIMES   YES
4. Do you feel handicapped by a hearing problem?
   NO   SOMETIMES   YES
5. Does a hearing problem cause you difficulty when visiting
   friends, relatives, or neighbors?
   NO   SOMETIMES   YES
6. Does a hearing problem cause you to attend religious services
   less often than you would like?
   NO   SOMETIMES   YES
7. Does a hearing problem cause you to have arguments with
   family members?
   NO   SOMETIMES   YES
8. Does a hearing problem cause you difficulty when listening to
   television or radio?
   NO   SOMETIMES   YES
9. Do you feel that any difficulty with your hearing limits or
   hampers your personal or social life?
   NO   SOMETIMES   YES
10. Does a hearing problem cause you difficulty when in a restau-
    rant with relatives or friends?
    NO   SOMETIMES   YES

1. Ask the patient to follow your finger with his eyes as it moves laterally in the visual field and to hold laterally but not in extreme lateral gaze.
2. Observe for end-point vacillation (nystagmus) of the globes.

For the comatose patient, caloric testing would be used in the extended examination.

Interpretation.

1. Unilateral or recent change by history in hearing acuity may be seen in disease of the auditory canal, tympanic membrane, ossicles of the middle ear, CN VIII, or the cerebral cortex. Definition of the anatomical location and etiology of the problem requires sorting out, some of which can be done with the relatively simple bedside maneuvers discussed below.
2. Vestibular dysfunction, based on either history of vertigo or discovery of nystagmus on screening, demands detailed neurologic history and physical examination before deciding on subsequent diagnostic steps. The lesion may be local (as in labyrinthitis), systemic (as in drug or alcohol intoxication), or central (as in cerebellar or brainstem disorders).

HEARING HANDICAP INVENTORY FOR THE ELDERLY

Goal. Screen further for functionally significant hearing loss.

Technique. Administer the inventory.

Interpretation. Each "no" answer represents 4 points, each "sometimes" answer represents 2 points, and each "yes" answer represents 6 points. A total of 8 points establishes probable hearing loss; a total of 24 or more points indicates certain hearing loss.

RINNE AND WEBER TESTS

Goal. Differentiate neurosensory from conductive hearing loss.

Technique. *Rinne test.* Set a 512-cycles/second tuning fork in motion. Hold the base of the fork against one mastoid process, and ask the patient to signal when he can no longer hear the hum. At this signal, move the vibrating fork near the external auditory meatus on the same side, and ask the patient whether he still hears the sound. If the patient hears the hum conducted through the auditory canal (air) after it has disappeared from the mastoid (bone) placement, he has a normal Rinne test; i.e., air conduction is better than bone conduction. If the patient *cannot* hear air-transmitted sound after its disappearance from bone placement, he has an abnormal Rinne test; i.e., air conduction is poorer than bone conduction. The test is then performed on the opposite ear and mastoid.

Weber test. Holding the base of the vibrating tuning fork on the midline of the forehead, ask the patient to indicate where he perceives sound. A normal response is "in the middle" or "all over." If it is louder in one ear than the other, the Weber test is lateralized and abnormal.

Interpretation. For use of these two tests to distinguish conductive from sensorineural hearing loss, see Table 4.3.

Table 4.3
Rinne and Weber Test Results Interpretation[a]

Description	Rinne	Weber
Left ear, pure sensorineural	AC > BC	Lateralizes to right
Right ear, normal	AC > BC	
Left ear, pure conductive loss	BC > AC	Lateralizes to left
Right ear, normal	AC > BC	
Left ear, mixed deafness	Cannot predict	Cannot predict
Right ear, normal	AC > BC	
Bilateral sensorineural deafness		
Left ear	AC > BC	Lateralizes to better
Right ear	AC > BC	(less diseased) ear
Bilateral conductive loss		
Left ear	BC > AC	Lateralizes to worse
Right ear	BC > AC	(more diseased) ear
Bilateral mixed deafness	Cannot predict any test results	

[a]AC, air conduction; and BC, bone conduction.

CALORIC TESTING OF THE COMATOSE PATIENT

Goal. Assess brainstem function.
Technique.
1. Use otoscopy to check that tympanic membranes are not perforated.
2. Keep the patient supine, with the patient's trunk at 30° to the bed.
3. Irrigate the external auditory canal via a syringe with 250 ml of water at 7°cooler than body temperature (30°C).
4. Observe for nystagmus; note whether it beats toward or away from the irrigated side.
5. Repeat with warmed water at 44°C.
Interpretation.
1. Nystagmus occurring toward warm water and away from cold water is normal.
2. Absence of response to both indicates canal paresis. Repeat the test with ice water to establish interpretable results.
3. Unilateral failure to respond indicates that the central connections of CN VIII are impaired.

Cranial Nerves IX and X:
Glossopharyngeal and Vagus

Goal. Assess sensory branch of CN IX and motor branch of CN X.
Technique.
1. With the patient's mouth open and the light shining against the palate and posterior pharynx, ask him to say "hat" long and loud. Observe the palate for symmetrical elevation.
2. Touch each side of the posterior pharynx with the tip of a cotton swab. Observe for symmetrical contraction of the pharynx.
3. Listen to phonation.
4. Observe deglutition of a sip of water.

Interpretation.
1. Failure of one side of the palate to elevate suggests a unilateral CN X lesion.
2. Absence of any gag reflex may be a normal variant; it can also be seen in many acute neurologic and systemic diseases. Failure of one side of the pharynx to contract with stimulus also indicates unilateral CN X abnormality.
3. Aberrant phonation may partake of CN IX-X dysfunction.
4. Delayed or difficult swallowing or nasal regurgitation strongly implicates CN IX-X dysfunction.

Cranial Nerve XI

Cranial nerve XI is discussed in Chapter 5, Neck.

Cranial Nerve XII: Hypoglossal

Goal. Assess integrity of the motor nerve to the tongue.
Technique.
1. Ask the patient to protrude his tongue forward. Observe for deviation from midline.
2. Ask the patient to push his tongue forcefully against your finger through each cheek. Assess for asymmetry in force.

Interpretation.
1. Deviation of the tongue on forward protrusion suggests unilateral disease of CN XII on the side toward which the tongue deviates, i.e., failure of ipsilateral "pushing power."
2. Asymmetry of power indicates a lesion of the nerve or brainstem in the cheek with weaker protrusion.
3. Hemiatrophy or fasciculation of the tongue muscle strongly suggests neurologic disease affecting CN XII on the affected side.

5

Neck

GENERAL ASSESSMENT OF NECK

Goal. Seek gross structural or positional abnormalities (see Figs. 5.1 and 5.2).

Technique. Standing directly in front of the patient, inspect for the following:

- Is the head held straight and comfortably?
- Are major muscles symmetrical?
- Is the trachea midline?
- Are there skin abnormalities or lesions?

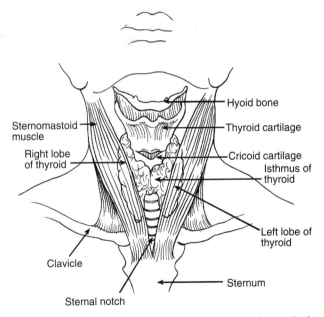

Figure 5.1 Relative positions of the bones near the trachea and of cartilages of the trachea and their relationships to the thyroid gland.

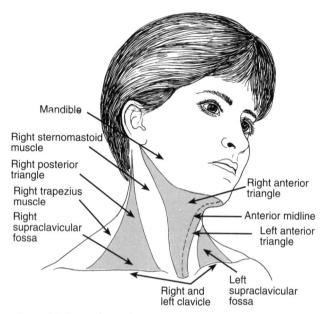

Figure 5.2 Cervical triangles.

Interpretation. If there are any asymmetries or abnormalities, perform an extended examination of the specific structure (see below). If the patient has a short, webbed neck, consider *Klippel-Feil anomaly*, congenital fusion of cervical vertebrae, and *Turner's syndrome* (XO karyotype).

Torticollis refers to a twisting of the neck secondary to spasm or disease of the muscles controlling the cervical spine. When acute, this is considered to be the result of inflammation, either viral or traumatic. Phenothiazines may also cause acute "wryneck," usually accompanied by other symptoms such as abnormal movements.

"NECK SIGN"

Goal. Look for the "neck sign" as part of the assessment for systemic sclerosis.

Technique.
1. Have the patient stand or sit in a relaxed position with arms dropped to the sides.
2. Have the patient extend the head with the chin pointing forward and up.
3. Look for tightness and ridging on the longitudinal skin folds of the patient's neck.
4. If ridges are found, palpate them to determine if they are lax or taut.

Interpretation. The neck sign is positive if tight, hard cords form on the skin surface with the neck extended. A positive sign suggests scleroderma. Normal aged persons may have soft cords.

CERVICAL SPINE

Goal. Assess the anatomical and functional status of the cervical spine.

Technique.
1. Observe the curve of the spine in lateral view.
2. Ask the patient to move the head into six positions: hyperextension, lateral flexion to right and left, anterior flexion, side-to-side rotation (Fig. 5.3).
3. Percuss the spinous processes.

Interpretation.
- Normal gentle extension curve
  1. Variations may be related to old trauma or surgery
  2. Anterior compression fractures may cause the head and neck to be thrust forward, as may spondylosis
- Abnormalities of movement
  1. Limitation of movement in any plane without pain
        Osteoarthrosis, flexion often most severely limited
        Voluntary for fear of precipitating pain
        Voluntary as psychologic symptom, malingering
  2. Limitation of movement in any plane with pain
        Osteoarthrosis
        Inflammatory arthritides (e.g., rheumatoid)
        Cervical disc disease
        Other local conditions, including torticollis

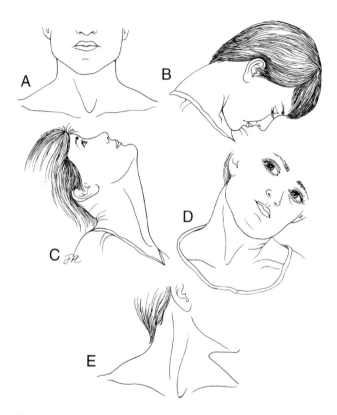

Figure 5.3 Normal cervical spine range of motion. **A.** Resting motion.
B. Anterior flexion. **C**. Extension. **D.** Lateral flexion ("tipping") to left.
E. Lateral rotation to left.

   3. Tenderness to percussion
           Over specific spinous process or facet joint
           Cervical spondylosis
           Osteomyelitis or paraspinal abscess

Special Maneuvers for Study of the Cervical Spine

COMPRESSION TEST

Goal. Evaluate for joint pain as the etiology of neck pain.

Technique.
1. Have the patient flex the head laterally toward the painful side and extend the neck slightly.
2. Place steady pressure downward on the head, thus compressing the ipsilateral articular pillar.

Interpretation. Sharply localized pain may define anatomical location of the pathologic process, usually *nonarticular.*

QUADRANT TEST

Goal. Evaluate for joint pain as the etiology of neck pain.

Technique.
1. Have the patient flex the head laterally toward the painful side, extend the neck slightly, and actively rotate the head toward the painful side.
2. Place steady pressure downward on the head.

Interpretation. As with the compression test, a positive quadrant test with a negative compression test localizes the problem to the intervertebral foramina.

Cervical Spinal Root

Goal. Assess for cervical spinal nerve root disease.

Technique.
1. *C5:* Check sensation of the patient's upper arm and upper outer forearm, forceful abduction of the arms held at 45° to the vertical against resistance (deltoid muscle), and the biceps muscle.
2. *C6:* Check sensation over the palmar surface of the patient's thumb and index finger, flexion of the supinated forearm against resistance (biceps muscle), and brachioradialis reflex (C5-C6).

3. *C7:* Check sensation over the patient's middle finger, extension of the partially flexed elbow against resistance (triceps muscle), and triceps reflex (C6-C7-C8).
4. *C8:* Check sensation over the patient's fifth finger and extension of the wrist against resistance.
5. *C7-T1:* Check the patient's handgrip.

Interpretation. For nerve compression syndromes, refer to Chapter 10, Limbs.

BLOOD VESSELS

Goal. Assess for arterial occlusive disease.
Technique.
1. To discern bruits in the vertebral artery, hold the bell of the stethoscope to the lower posterior border of the sternomastoid.
2. To listen for bruits in the subclavian artery, press down and back into the supraclavicular fossa from the upper side of the posterior margin of the junction of the medial and middle thirds of the clavicle to locate pulsation. "Snuggle" the bell at this point. If an acoustic seal cannot be obtained, employ a pediatric bell.
3. To palpate the innominate artery-aorta complex, observe the jugular notch for pulsations and introduce a fingertip from above a bit inferiorly into the notch.

Interpretation. For discrimination among sounds in the neck, see Chapter 8, Heart and Great Vessels. Cervical venous hums are common in normal children and may also represent high cardiac output from pregnancy, cirrhosis, anemia, or hyperthyroidism. Continuous cervical murmur that abates when the patient reclines is usually a venous hum. Digital pressure over the superior aspect of the mid-clavicle should compress the external jugular vein and abrogate the sound. The Valsalva maneuver will often make a venous hum disappear, whereas active rotation of the neck away from the side being auscultated may intensify a venous hum. Systolic sound high in the neck may be a

carotid bruit. A sound that attenuates as the stethoscope is
inched up the neck from the root is likely a transmitted cardiac murmur.

THYROID GLAND

Goal. Assess the thyroid gland for size and masses.
Technique.
1. Instruct the patient to keep the head straight;
   observe for thyroid movement after the patient
   swallows a sip of water. Use strong cross-lighting.
   The patient's chin should not be elevated.
2. Palpate as follows (Fig. 5.4):
   a. Stand behind the seated patient, place the fingers
      of your right hand anterior to the patient's right
      sternomastoid, and press forward and medially
      against the right lateral trachea.
   b. With the fingers of your left hand, compress the
      left lobe of the gland from the front.
   c. Ask the patient to swallow a sip of water, and
      feel the left lobe move upward beneath your
      fingers.
   d. Palpate the lobe for consistency, nodularity, and
      tenderness.

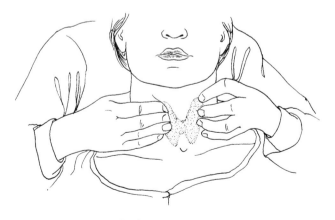

Figure 5.4 Thyroid gland palpation.

    e. Reverse hand placement to assess the right lobe.
    f. To feel the isthmus, place two fingers of each hand over the patient's lower tracheal cartilage and palpate for the soft band of glandular tissue.
    g. If a nodule or nodules are felt, estimate their size, character, and location (upper pole, middle, lower pole).

Problem solving. If the sternomastoids seem tight and are obscuring palpation, have the patient try to flex the neck laterally *slightly* toward the side being examined. If the neck is thick, have the patient try to extend the neck slightly and clasp hands behind the neck.

Interpretation. Each lobe of a normal thyroid gland is 4–5 cm in height and 2 cm wide. The right lobe is often slightly larger than the left. The thyroid is commonly not palpable in adults. The gland enlarges slightly during adolescence and pregnancy. Interpretation of some findings follows:

1. A full-looking lower neck that fails to rise with swallowing is usually nonthyroidal, e.g., muscle and fat. Rarely, it may indicate Riedel's thyroiditis or fixed thyroid cancer.
2. Tenderness on palpation suggests thyroiditis.
3. Lymphadenopathy in the presence of diffuse thyroid enlargement may indicate the lymphoid hyperplasia of Graves' hyperthyroidism or, less commonly, metastatic thyroid carcinoma.
4. Low-pitched sounds heard directly over the thyroid that disappear with pressure on the bell are usually generated in the gland, classically in diffuse toxic hyperplasia (Graves' disease).

CERVICAL LYMPH NODES

Goal. Discover enlargement of or unusual consistency in the cervical lymph nodes (see Figs. 5.5 and 5.6).

Technique. Face the patient and palpate both sides of the patient's neck simultaneously, using the pads and tips of your three middle fingers held at 45° to the skin plane.

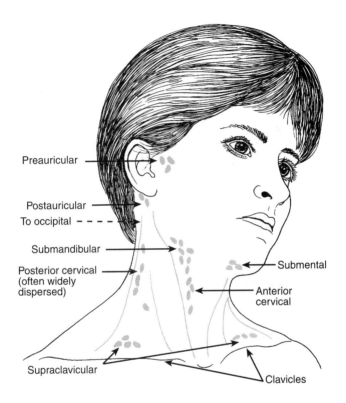

Preauricular
Postauricular
To occipital
Submandibular
Posterior cervical (often widely dispersed)
Supraclavicular
Submental
Anterior cervical
Clavicles

Figure 5.5 Surface projections of the chains of cervical lymph nodes.

Maintain contact with the skin while moving the fingers in small circles along each chain in the following order:

1. Begin with the postauricular and preauricular groups.
2. Move to the angle of the jaw and palpate along the inferior rami of the mandible.
3. Move to the occiput and palpate the posterior triangle behind the sternomastoid; then move inferiorly to the lateral retroclavicular area.
4. Move laterally to the supraclavicular fossae.

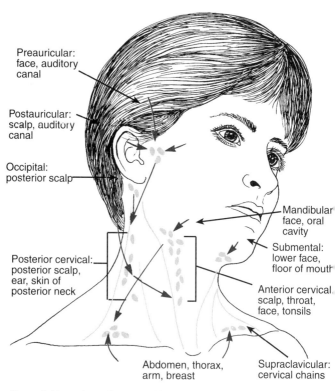

Preauricular:
face, auditory
canal

Postauricular:
scalp, auditory
canal

Occipital:
posterior scalp

Posterior cervical:
posterior scalp,
ear, skin of
posterior neck

Mandibular
face, oral
cavity

Submental:
lower face,
floor of mouth

Anterior cervical:
scalp, throat,
face, tonsils

Abdomen, thorax,
arm, breast

Supraclavicular:
cervical chains

Figure 5.6 Lymphatic drainage of head and neck.

5. Begin at the angle of the jaw and palpate anterior triangles along the anterior border of the sternomastoid down to its attachment at the clavicles.

Problem solving. For the most intensive search of the supraclavicular fossae, use any one or all of the following:

1. Palpate from behind with flexed fingers curled over the patient's shoulder (Fig. 5.7).
2. Have the patient perform the Valsalva maneuver.
3. Repeat the examination with the patient supine, positioning yourself at the head of the table.

Interpretation.

- Enlarged lymph nodes
    1. Submandibular—may be salivary gland ptosis
    2. Occipital—local (scalp) infection; also can be part of generalized lymphadenopathy
- Hard nodes as markers for potential cancer metastases (see also Fig. 5.6)
    1. Submandibular—cancer of nose, lip, anterior tongue, anterior floor of the mouth
    2. Middle jugular—cancer of base of tongue or larynx
    3. Lower jugular—cancer of thyroid or cervical esophagus
    4. High posterior cervical—cancer of nasopharynx
    5. Left supraclavicular (Virchow)—cancer of stomach, esophagus, left lung, or other abdominal or pelvic cancers
    6. Right supraclavicular—cancer of right lung, *base* of left lung, abdominal organs
- Generalized lymphadenopathy

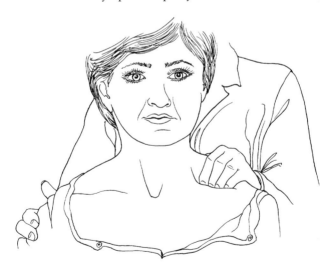

Figure 5.7 Palpation of supraclavicular lymph nodes.

1. Hematologic malignancies, especially lymphomas and chronic lymphocytic leukemia
2. HIV infection with progressive generalized lymph-adenopathy
3. Other viral illnesses, especially Epstein-Barr virus and cytomegalovirus
4. Mycobacterioses and other granulomatous infections
5. Syphilis or toxoplasmosis
6. Immune-stimulated lymphoid hyperplasia, e.g., Graves' disease
7. Phenytoin therapy
8. Sarcoidosis

- Massive cervical lymph nodes
  1. Hematologic malignancies
  2. Reactive hyperplasia
  3. Solid neoplasms with unusually large metastases
  4. Proliferative HIV lymphadenopathy
- Soft fluctuant nodes
  1. Necrosis with suppuration, usually bacterial in etiology
  2. Cat-scratch disease
  3. Spontaneous necrosis in cancer metastasis
- Nodes fixed to skin or other tissue
  1. Tuberculosis, e.g., scrofula
  2. Malignant neoplasia
  3. Aggressive infective inflammation

CERVICAL MASSES

Goal. Evaluate lumps in the neck.
Technique.
1. In a darkened room, try to transilluminate the mass with a bright, narrow beam (penlight, flashlight apposed to skin at back of mass).
2. Watch and feel for elevation of the mass as patient sticks out tongue.
3. Observe the effect of swallowing. Does the mass move?
4. Watch the mass while the patient blows hard through pursed lips for 10 seconds. Does the mass enlarge?

5. Watch what happens when the patient performs the Valsalva maneuver.
6. Assess for attachment to the sternomastoid muscle:
   a. Have the patient lie supine with a pillow beneath the head.
   b. Then have the patient lift the head 4 cm from the pillow and rotate the neck away from the lump.
   c. Observe whether the mass is visibly attached to or continuous with the contracted muscle.

Interpretation (see Fig. 5.8).

1. A mass that transilluminates may be a cystic hygroma or a diverticulum arising from any cervical segment of the upper aerodigestive tract.
2. A mass that rises when the tongue is protruded is likely to be a thyroglossal duct cyst.
3. A mass that elevates with swallowing is almost always thyroidal.
4. Blowing through pursed lips enlarges a laryngocele.
5. The Valsalva maneuver enlarges a laryngocele or a jugular venous ectasia.
6. Attachment to the sternomastoid suggests *(a)* fixation from inflammation, *(b)* neoplasm, or *(c)* origin from the muscle itself, e.g., fibroma.

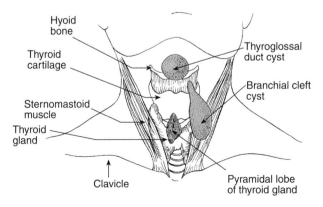

Figure 5.8 Surface projections of several cervical masses.

TRACHEA

Goal. Assess for deviation, tenderness, or abnormal motion of the trachea.

Technique.
1. Look at the patient's trachea in the suprasternal notch. Is it deviated from midline? With your finger tips, locate the hyoid bone, then move downward to the larger thyroid cartilage. Are all structures midline or symmetric?
2. Is there tenderness to palpation?
3. To assess for tracheal tug, have the patient sit down, with mouth closed and chin fully elevated. Hold the cricoid cartilage between your thumb and index finger and press upward.
4. Auscultate the trachea for wheezing.

Interpretation.
1. Deviation of the trachea occurs *toward* atelectatic lung and fibrosis but *away from* large pleural effusions, pneumothoraces, or consolidations.
2. Tracheal tenderness is characteristic of nonpyogenic ("atypical") pneumonias.
3. Tracheal tug, a systolic downward-inward pull on the fingers through expiration, means the aorta is tethered to the bronchial system and the attached airway is transmitting aortic pulsations.
4. Tracheal wheezes can mean turbulent flow from partial obstruction of the upper airway or from propagation of lower airway noise. Purely inspiratory wheezes are stridorous and indicate a laryngotracheal origin.

CRANIAL NERVE XI

Goal. Assess the integrity of cranial nerve XI and the trapezii and sternomastoids that it innervates.

Technique.
1. Place your hands on top of the medial part of the patient's shoulders and ask the patient to shrug both shoulders. Shoulders should rise symmetrically, and

contracted muscle mass should be symmetrical (Fig. 5.9).

2. Ask the patient to rotate the head to the right. Then, while you place your right palm against the patient's left mandibular ramus, ask the patient to rotate the head leftward against the resistance of your palm. This tests the left sternomastoid. Reverse the procedure to test the right.

Interpretation. These muscles are normally symmetrical in position, size, and strength. Any deviation from symmetry signifies either disease of the muscle body or loss of cranial nerve XI function.

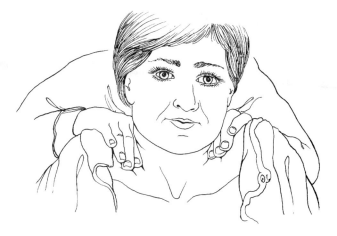

Figure 5.9 Testing cranial nerve XI—shoulder shrug component. Shrug is against the examiner's downward pressure.

6

Breasts and Axillae

Goals.
1. Detect threatening breast and lymph node diseases—prototypically **breast cancer**—to secure timely intervention.
2. Reassure women who are free of serious breast disease, and enhance behaviors that optimize lifetime early detection.
3. Address the high anxiety level about this area: most women equate breast problems with cancer and regard this with terror.

Technique. *Timing.* Whenever possible, breast examination in reproductive age women is conducted soon after the end of menses.

Ask routine breast-related questions before initiating the physical examination, lest the patient fear that an abnormal finding has occasioned the query.

History taking. Take a history of **mass** or other breast problems, prior breast biopsies or cancers, breast pain, nipple changes or discharge, breast trauma, date of the last menstrual period, and possibility of pregnancy. If the issue is nipple secretion, ask about *(a)* the use of estrogens, tricyclic antidepressants, phenothiazines, and some antihypertensives; *(b)* endocrine problems such as hyperthyroidism, hypothalamic or pituitary tumors, Cushing's syndrome, or known hyperprolactinemia; and *(c)* unusual breast stimulation (in men also) and androgenic symptoms such as increased facial hair, libido, clitoral size, recurrent acne, or change in menstrual pattern.

Inspection. Inspect the chest with the patient seated, with both arms and both sides of the chest fully exposed. Modesty must be subordinated to the vital diagnostic role that is incompatible with it. Inspect the integument, nipple, and areola contour. Know the expected breast contour for developmental stage (Fig. 6.1).

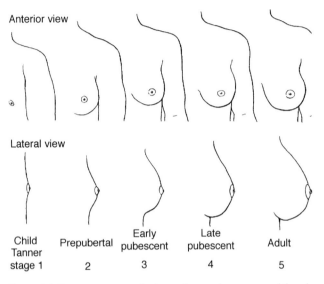

Figure 6.1 Tanner stage terminology of normal sequence of female breast development.

Look at the effect of movement. As the patient raises her arms above her head, observe for symmetry of breast and nipple motion and for end-position (Fig. 6.2*A*). Watch for dimpling of the skin, deviation of a nipple, or change in skin contour. Have the patient place her hands on her waist and press inward (Fig. 6.2*B*). Also have her put her hands behind her head and pull her elbows forward. Ask any patient with very large or pendulous breasts to lean forward from the waist, and observe for an asymmetric or locally altered effect of this gravitational pull (Fig. 6.2*C*).

Examine the axillae. Inspect each axilla by having the patient raise her arm over her head. Firm, continuous skin contact during palpation will help to minimize pain or tick-lishness. For the patient's left axilla, slide your right hand upward along the midaxillary chest wall until the humerus

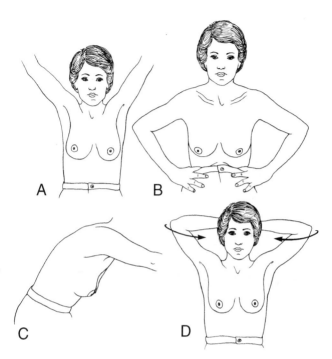

Figure 6.2 Four positions to observe the breasts for asymmetry on movement, skin dimpling or retraction, or nipple deviation. **A.** Arms elevated over head. **B.** Hands pressing on hips with pectoralis muscles tensed. **C.** Leaning forward with breast tissue dependent. **D.** Hands clasped behind head to accomplish tensing of pectoralis major muscles.

is met. From high in the axilla, palpate downward along the border of the pectoralis muscle with the palmar surface of your fingers, compressing the tissue against the chest wall to about the level of the nipple (anterior axillary chain). Returning to the apex of the axilla, repeat the maneuver at the posterior extremity of the axillary hollow, i.e., along the anterior border of the latissimus dorsi muscle (subscapular chain). Reversing the hand such that the palmar surface lies against the humerus, search for the subhumeral nodes. Use your left hand to repeat these maneuvers in the patient's right axilla.

When axillary lymphadenopathy is found, evaluate all structures that drain into it, not just the breast. Ask about cat scratches, and inspect the ipsilateral hand and forearm for inflammation and the axilla for infected hair follicles.

Palpate the breasts. With the patient supine and draped, as you stand on her right, each breast is exposed and palpated individually. The patient places each arm, in turn, under her head as the ipsilateral breast is examined. If the breast is large, a small towel is folded under the same shoulder to spread breast tissue further across the chest wall.

Effective breast palpation requires a systematic sequence (Fig. 6.3), e.g.,

- The "back-and-forth" technique in rows from superior to inferior
- The "quadrantic" method, particularly useful for small breasts with little pendulous tissue
  Additional pointers for breast palpation are
- Utilize the pads of the fingers, not the tips.
- Maintain continuous skin contact as the fingers move over the surface.
- Gently compress the breast tissue between the examining fingers and underlying chest wall structures. The ribs and cartilage of a very thin woman must be discriminated from breast mass.
- The motion of the fingers is that of "rolling" the mobile underlying tissue.
- The nipple and areola are palpated as discrete structures by pressing them against the chest wall. Tell the patient that some pressing of the nipple is required. Gently compress the areola at the base of the nipple between your thumb and forefinger. The tissue is "milked" toward the surface of the nipple to express any fluid present within the ducts. Any nipple secretion recov-ered in this manner is inspected and characterized by color, viscosity, and lat-erality. A clean glass slide can be pressed directly against any secretion on the nipple and sprayed immediately with fixative for a *Papanicolaou smear*. If there is heat, tenderness, purulent discharge, or other indication of infection, a smear can be *Gram-stained* and sent for culture.

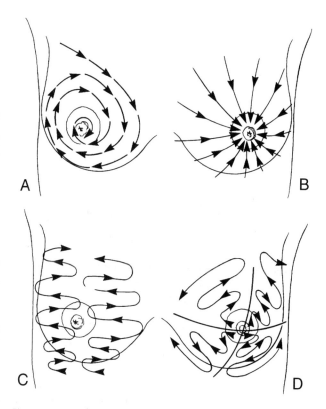

Figure 6.3 Four alternative methods for systematic palpation of breast. **A.** Spiral, beginning with the tail. **B.** Spokes, centripetally. **C.** Back-and-forth method. **D.** Quadrantic, i.e., palpation of each quadrant, centrifugally.

• To effect adequate spread of the large breast for thorough palpation of the outer quadrants, have the patient cup her hand under the dependent tissue and hold it medially.

The male breast. Routinely inspect and palpate the male breast with the patient in the sitting position. If the breasts are large, employ techniques as for a woman.

Breast mass evaluation. Thoroughly palpate the nonin-volved breast and the uninvolved quadrants of the abnor-mal side to establish background consistency and density. Then determine and record the following:

- Size of the mass in its vertical and horizontal dimen-sions, measured with a ruler or tape measure.
- Location by quadrant and by distance from the areolar rim.
- Consistency, such as compressible or cystic, firm or rock-hard.
- Shape and character of edges, e.g., round, elliptical, or diffuse and ill-defined.
- Character of the overlying skin (increased temperature, erythema, edema, retraction).
- Attachment of mass to overlying skin or subjacent fascia, muscle, or chest wall or the absence of fixation. Does the area move freely with the rest of the breast, remain stationary, or retract as the patient raises her arms over her head? When she tenses the pectoralis muscles by pressing hands on hips or clasping them behind her back, does the abnormal area move differ-ently from the remainder of the breast?

Interpretation. *Visible attributes.* The shape, size, and symmetry of female breasts vary widely. Visible difference in size between the two breasts is the rule rather than the exception.

Pigmentation of the areola varies with general skin pig-mentation and tends to darken during pregnancy and retain the darker coloration permanently. The areola is normally dotted with tiny papular structures, the sebaceous glands of Montgomery, with variable prominence.

Rudimentary nipples (polythelia) and small supernu-merary breasts (polymastia) may normally be discovered along the "milk line" from each anterior axilla to the proxi-mal medial thigh.

The venous pattern of the breasts is accentuated during normal pregnancy and lactation. At other times, and espe-cially if asymmetric, consider an underlying tumor. Palpate the tissue deep to any suspicious skin abnormality. Is there induration beneath the skin? Is there a mass? The absence of a mass does not rule out cancer, nor does the presence of one necessarily signify cancer.

Acute *mastitis* characteristically produces *unilateral breast enlargement* and occurs during lactation. The involved tissue is red, indurated, and exquisitely tender. *Inflammatory carcinoma* of the breast can mimic mastitis. As with Paget's disease of the breast, the absence of a subjacent breast mass offers no reassurance. *Congestive heart failure* with consistent lateral recumbency can produce unilateral breast enlargement.

Nipple characteristics and secretion. Adult nipples are normally everted symmetrically. Acquired inversion or flattening demands further investigation. Even without a palpable mass in the area, it is presumed cancerous.

The nipple is subject to irritation by clothing fabrics, to contact dermatitis, and to fissure, especially with breast-feeding. Paget's disease of the breast is a form of carcinoma that causes crusting and erosion of the nipple or areola. Apparent eczema of the breast must always be viewed with suspicion even without a palpable subjacent mass.

During pregnancy, the breasts may secrete colostrum on minimal stimulation. As pregnancy advances, the clear discharge becomes more viscous and slightly yellowish. Except during pregnancy and lactation, nipple secretion is considered abnormal, although *sometimes* no cause is found.

Breast texture. The elongated segment of the upper outer quadrant, which extends in some women high along the border of the pectoralis muscle, is the tail of the breast (tail of Spence). The inferior border of the breast often contains a crescent or thick line of palpably dense fibrous tissue, the **inframammary ridge.**

The consistency of normal breasts varies greatly. The normal breast in an adult woman of reproductive age who is neither pregnant nor lactating is coarsely granular and uniform in consistency. The so-called fibrocystic breast is a normal variant, but it may present recurrent diagnostic problems. Once menstrual cycling is established, the normal breast can become tense, slightly swollen, and tender during the secretory phase, especially in the week preceding menstruation, with increase in palpable fibrocystic components.

During pregnancy, the breasts enlarge and become lobular, even multinodular. If breast-feeding is undertaken, the breasts remain firm and enlarged for the duration of lactation.

After menopause, the glandular tissue of the breast atrophies, and the breast may appear elongated and flattened and feel more uniform, more finely granular, and softer than before. Fibrocystic changes, if occurring, tend to regress in both extent and distinctness.

Breast masses. Any new mass, even in the setting of underlying fibrocystic tissue, is suspicious for cancer, although many turn out to be other processes.

Retraction or asymmetrical movement suggests fixation of the skin to underlying tissue—usually a feature of locally advanced cancer—as does nipple deviation of the involved breast with arm-raising.

- *Discrete, nontender masses*

    The common **benign cyst** is typically round to slightly elliptical, soft and elastic, and freely mobile. There is fixation or retraction. Although usually nontender, cysts may become tender prior to menses. Cysts are often multiple and bilateral and are commonly symmetric both within a breast and between breasts. They often vary in size with the menstrual cycle, being smallest just after menses. For the experienced surgeon, needle aspiration with cytologic study of the fluid often secures the diagnosis and corrects the problem all at once.

    Fibroadenoma is a benign solid mass that may appear any time after puberty but presents less commonly after menopause. It is usually solitary. Like the cyst, it is well demarcated, freely mobile, usually nontender, and never fixed.

    Cancer of the breast may present at any age after puberty; the likelihood that a mass will turn out to be cancerous increases progressively with age. Characteristically, the late **breast cancer** is irregular, very firm to hard, and not clearly delineated from surrounding tissue. *These features are not uniformly present, however, particularly in earlier lesions, and their absence does not exclude cancer.* Although fixation to skin and to the chest wall occur in advanced disease, early carcinomas—those one most wants to discover—seldom have retraction signs. Similarly, although cancers are usually painless, tenderness of a breast lesion does not exclude malignancy.

Less common nontender solitary masses include fat necrosis, idiopathic granulomatous mastitis, tuberculosis of the breast, and giant cell arteritis.

- *Discrete, tender masses*

    Acute *abscess* of the breast is well-localized, hot, tender, and often fluctuant. It is frequently accompanied by fever and chills and may follow acute mastitis, typically during lactation.

    With a less erythematous and hot area, consider *galactocele*, the cystic dilation caused by duct blockage in the lactating breast. This soft mass usually disappears upon use of a breast pump to enhance drainage.

    Male breast findings. A small disc of fibrofatty tissue is felt directly under the areola in many adolescent boys and some men. With obesity, fat can accumulate beneath the areola, giving the visual impression of gynecomastia. Palpation usually discloses whether the enlargement is glandular (gynecomastic), adipose, or suspicious for tumor.

    Exogenous estrogen, such as in the treatment of prostatic carcinoma, regularly produces **gynecomastia**; other causes include adrenal and testicular malfunction, cirrhosis, and the effects of some drugs including digoxin.

    A visible or palpable subareolar mass, nipple retraction, or secretion may represent male breast cancer. Male breast cancer is often diagnosed at an advanced stage because of failure to consider the possibility as well as anatomic factors.

    Axillary lymphadenopathy. Very hard, fixed, or matted nodes in the axilla are highly suggestive of cancer but are a late sign, so the lack of this sign is not reassuring that a breast mass is benign. If small, slightly tender, mobile, soft axillary lymph nodes are found unilaterally, consider not only breast cancer but also inflammatory conditions.

Substantial bilateral axillary lymphadenopathy suggests a systemic stimulus to lymphoid hyperplasia, or primary lymphoid neoplasia, or the effects of bilateral breast cancer.

7

Thorax and Lungs

General observation of a patient suspected of having chronic lung disease may provide clues such as

- **Cyanosis:** Indicative of oxygen desaturation
- **Pursed lips:** Indicative of expiratory difficulty
- **Position signs of severe obstructive pulmonary disease**
    Professorial position: Leaning forward, bracing trunk with arms and hands
    Seated position, with elbows on knees and head in hands
    Seated sleep
- **Dahl's sign** (calluses or hyperkeratotic areas on anterior thigh just above knees): From staying in the seated position for very protracted periods

CHEST WALL OBSERVATION (FIGS. 7.1–7.3)

Goal. Assess structure and motion of the chest wall.

Technique. Systematically observe the front, back, and side of the patient's thorax.

Frontal view. Facing the patient, look for *(a)* shape and symmetry of the bony thorax, *(b)* rate and rhythm of respiration, *(c)* ease of respiration, *(d)* retraction of respiratory muscles, and *(e)* symmetry of movement. Is the trachea midline? Is the trachea tender?

Lateral and posterior views. Standing at the patient's side, have the patient raise his arms over his head; look for thoracic configuration, including curves of the spine. Repeat the observation, standing behind the patient.

View from head of table. If there is a question of **asymmetry of movement,** stand at the head of the table and observe the patient in a supine position as he takes a deep breath. Does the abdomen protrude as the diaphragm descends and retract with expiration? Is there "off-the-top"

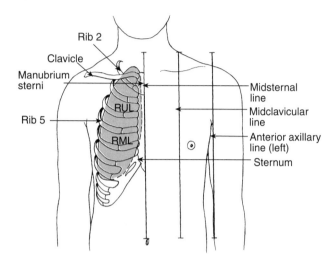

Figure 7.1 Surface projections of thoracic bone structures and pulmonary lobes with placement of anterior thoracic lines.

breathing in which inspiration begins without a full expiratory antecedent? Are the breaths shallow and panting from a respiratory midposition?

Chest expansion. Measure **chest expansion** with a tape measure: Subtract the circumference at full expiration from that at full inspiration.

Interpretation. *Chest.*

- *Shape:* **Barrel chest** may indicate air-trapping of airway obstruction but is also seen with anterior compression fractures and in the normal elderly. **Pectus excavatum** and **pectus carinatum** may be either congenital anomalies or the result of childhood vitamin D deficiency.

- *Rate and rhythm:* The normal adult *rate* is between 10 and 18 cycles/minute. **Tachypnea** is >18 cycles/minute, while **bradypnea** is <10 cycles/minute. *Rhythm* is normally regular, with expiration slightly longer than inspiration. **Hyperpnea,** which is rapid, deep respirations, suggests hyperventilation, acidosis, or pulmonary disease.

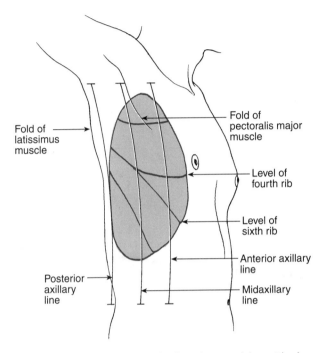

Figure 7.2 Surface projections of right pulmonary lobes with placement of lateral thoracic lines.

- *Ease of respiration:* Normally quiet, expiration passive.
- *Use of accessory muscles:* Should not be visible; if it is visible, obstructive rather than restrictive lung disease is more likely.
- *Asymmetry of movement:* The side with decreased movement is the more abnormal side.

Thoracic spine. Pathologic **kyphosis** commonly results from osteopenia and anterior vertebral collapse. **Scoliosis,** lateral curvature of the spine, may cause lung compression and restrictive respiratory disease.

Abnormal movement. **Absence of abdominal movement** indicates peritoneal pain or abdominal distension. **Complete abdominal respiratory movement** without tho-

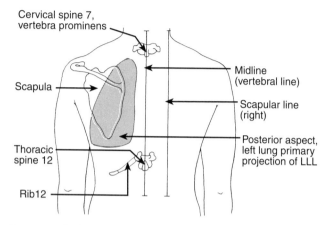

Figure 7.3 Surface projections of posterior pulmonary viscera with placement of posterior thoracic lines. LLL. left lower lobe.

racic motion is seen in lung or chest wall disease particularly when accompanied by pleuritic pain. **Abdominothoracic dyssynchrony** (abdominal wall retraction during inspiration) indicates a weak or paralyzed hemidiaphragm from unilateral phrenic nerve palsy, muscle disease, or respiratory overwork. **Respiratory alternans** consists of a few normal breaths alternating with a few of dyssynergy, reflecting temporary exhaustion of the diaphragm.

Chest expansion. Decreased chest expansion may be seen with disease of chest wall, pleura, lungs, or dorsal spine.

PALPATION AND PERCUSSION OF BONY THORAX

Goal. Seek skeletal disease of the thorax or assess chest pain.

Technique.
1. To elicit spinal tenderness, percuss over each dorsal vertebral spinous process with the ulnar surface of your fist.
2. **Springing a rib** can be used to seek a suspected fracture; i.e., press hard against a rib 15 cm from the suspected fracture.

3. To test for **costochondritis,** press your fingertip firmly against each costochondral junction, 2 cm lateral to each sternal border.

Interpretation.

1. Spinal tenderness may indicate cancer, fresh fracture, or inflammatory disease.
2. A positive springing test of the rib consists of localized severe pain at a distance from the site compressed. It is diagnostic of rib fracture.
3. The finding of tender ribs suggests all the differential diagnoses of spinal tenderness and costochondritis. Point tenderness over one or more costochondral junctions strongly suggests costochondritis.

Palpation for Subcutaneous Emphysema

Goal. Seek evidence for air leakage from the respiratory system into the subcutis and, less commonly, assess swelling about the upper chest and neck.

Technique. Palpate gently for a "squishy" or popping sensation in the subcutis about the jugular notch, manubrium, clavicles, and supraclavicular fossae.

Interpretation. Soft popping without inflammatory skin signs suggests air leakage, as in pneumothorax with dissection out of the pleural space. When subcutaneous emphysema is combined with inflammatory signs (erythema, etc.), consider infection with gas-forming bacteria.

Costovertebral Angle Palpation

Goal. Assess for pyelonephritis.

Technique. Using a single finger, press firmly against each twelfth costovertebral angle (CVA), asking the patient to indicate any discomfort created by the pressure.

Interpretation. CVA tenderness, especially unilateral, suggests infection of the underlying kidney. A positive test may occur in tense persons, with perinephric inflammation, in some musculoskeletal strains, and in inflammatory processes of the spine.

PERCUSSION OF THE LUNG

Goal. Assess for lung parenchymal or pleural disease.

Technique. Indirect percussion consists of the following steps (Fig. 7.4):

1. Spread the palmar surfaces of the fingers of your one hand over the area to be percussed.

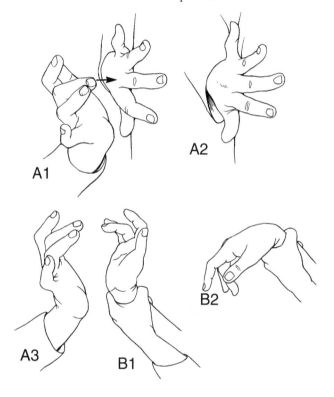

Figure 7.4 **A.** Chest wall percussion techniques. **A1.** Relative position of plexor and pleximeter at beginning of percussion stroke. **A2.** Pleximeter placement. **A3.** Plexor in position to begin percussion stroke. **B.** Practicing percussion, with fixation of wrist by opposite hand. **B1.** Full extension at beginning of stroke. **B2.** Full flexion at time of contact of plexor with pleximeter.

2. With the tip of the middle finger of your other hand *(plexor)*, strike the dorsum of distal interphalangeal (DIP) joint of the spread middle finger *(pleximeter)* quickly and sharply, with the wrist of the percussing hand used as the fulcrum of motion.

3. Note the sensation felt by the pleximeter and the sound created by the stroke.

Percussion of the Posterior and Lateral Lungs

For percussing the posterior and lateral lungs (Fig. 7.5), follow these steps:

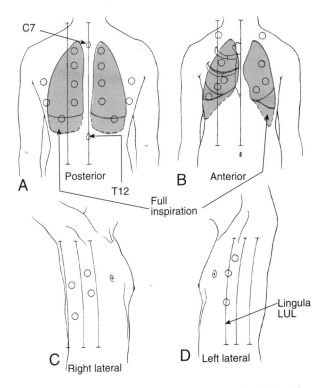

Figure 7.5 Sites for both percussion and auscultation marked with *circles*. LUL, left upper lobe.

1. Ask the patient to cross his arms across his chest to spread the scapulae.
2. Beginning high on the chest, percuss downward toward the base of each lung, assessing from side to side at symmetric points.
3. Move to the patient's right side and ask him to raise his right arm over his head.
4. Percuss from high in the axilla to the level of the diaphragm.
5. Move to the patient's left side and repeat the procedure.

Interpretation. For anticipated percussion notes over the adult thorax, see Figure 7.6. Interpretation of abnormal sounds follows:

• Unduly loud sounds on percussion

  Hyperresonance is common in pulmonary hyperinflation, as with asthma and chronic obstructive disease, and in patients with very thin chest walls, as in cachexia.

  Tympany is not encountered unless a large air pocket (bulla or pneumothorax) is separated from the pleximeter by a thin chest wall.

• Reduced sounds

  Dullness is heard with pulmonary disease or thick chest wall (obesity, extensive muscular development).

  Localized dullness is heard with consolidation of a portion of a lung.

  Flatness results from absence of contained air within the zone, as with pleural effusion or thick pleural scarring.

Percussion for Diaphragmatic Motion

Goal. Assess for limitations of hemidiaphragmatic motion.

Technique.

1. Ask the patient to take in full breath, exhale fully, and maintain full expiration. Percuss in the scapular line from about the T8 level until the note changes

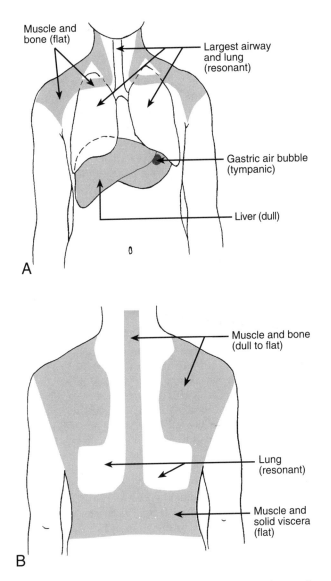

Muscle and
bone (flat)

Largest airway
and lung
(resonant)

Gastric air bubble
(tympanic)

Liver (dull)

A

Muscle and bone
(dull to flat)

Lung
(resonant)

Muscle and
solid viscera
(flat)

B

Figure 7.6 Normal percussion notes. **A.** Over anterior chest wall.
B. Over posterior chest wall. *White areas* represent resonance of pulmonary parenchyma; light-tinted areas, the dullness of non-air-filled
tissue; and dark-tinted area, the tympany of hollow viscera.

from resonance to dullness. With a skin pencil, mark the transition point on each hemithorax.
2. Ask the patient to take a deep breath and hold in full inspiration. Begin percussion downward in the scapular line, starting at the previously marked skin line, marking the new transition with a skin pencil.
3. Measure the distance between the two lines on each hemithorax; this is the *diaphragmatic excursion.*

Interpretation.
1. The right hemidiaphragm is normally slightly higher than the left.
2. Excursion of the normal leaf is ≥3 cm posteriorly.
3. Inability to detect a change in unilateral diaphragmatic position suggests phrenic nerve palsy as with a mediastinal mass or lung cancer. Large pleural effusions or large basal lung consolidation will obscure diaphragmatic excursion.

Percussion of the Apex

Goal. Seek apical consolidation as with tumor or infection.

Technique. Face the patient, rest your left hand at the root of the patient's neck, and drop your left thumb into the patient's right supraclavicular fossa as pleximeter. Strike the ulnar side of your thumb's interphalangeal joint with your plexor as above. For the left fossa, curl your hand around the back and left side of the patient's neck so that the tip of your left middle finger falls into the fossa and becomes the pleximeter. Strike the radial side of its DIP joint with the plexor.

Interpretation. Interpret the same as for Percussion of the Posterior and Lateral Lungs above, but if abnormalities are discovered, also consider tuberculosis and Pancoast tumor.

AUSCULTATION OF THE LUNGS

Goal. Assess air movement in large to medium-sized airways and make inferences about airways, parenchyma, and pleural space.

Technique.
1. Use the diaphragm of the stethoscope, warmed by rubbing it in the palm of your hand.
2. Ask the patient to breathe through open mouth.
3. Positioning of the stethoscope on the chest wall follows the same pattern as listed under Percussing the Posterior and Lateral Lungs: symmetric points, moving downward.
4. Compare breath sounds from side to side; assess each site through at least one full respiratory cycle.
5. Continue the procedure into each lateral hemithorax, positioning the instrument as for percussion.
6. Auscultate anterior lung fields from immediately below the clavicles to the level of the anterior diaphragmatic limits (Fig. 7.5*B*).

Interpretation. Expected breath sounds are **vesicular, bronchovesicular,** and **bronchial.** See Table 7.1 for characteristics of these sounds and Figure 7.6 for their locations.

Table 7.1
Normal Breath Sounds Heard on Auscultation

Sound	Quality	Location
Bronchial	Loud, pitch high, dominant in expiration	Trachea, anterior
Bronchovesicular	Medium volume and pitch, heard equally in inspiration and expiration	Main bronchi, anterior and some interscapular
Vesicular	Soft to medium, pitch lower dominant in inspiration	Over remainder of lung fields

Interpretation of these sounds follows:
- **Reduced breath sounds**
  Thick chest wall
  Reduced air flow, as in emphysema or with obstructed bronchus
  Interposition of fluid or air in pleural space, i.e., pleural effusion or pneumothorax
- **Increased and bronchial breath sounds**
  Normal over large airways

Consolidated air spaces, as in atelectasis, pneumonia, pulmonary edema

Replacement of alveolar air by scar tissue, granulomata, neoplasia

- **Prolonged expiration**

   Airway obstruction: mucus plugging, bronchial smooth-muscle spasm, inflammatory alteration

   Reduced lung elastic recoil: emphysema, old age

- **Wheezing**

   Markedly reduced airflow: bronchial obstruction, local or generalized as in asthmatic bronchospasm

- **Crackles** (rales)

   May be normal when very sparse and may be basilar in the elderly

   Persistent or new: atelectasis, fibrosis, inflammation, pulmonary edema, granuloma, tumor

   Purely early inspiratory crackles suggest severe obstructive airway disease; *paninspiratory* or purely late *inspiratory crackles* occur in all the lung diseases listed just above

- **Pleural rubs**

   Occur in both inspiration and expiration and sound like pieces of leather rubbing together

   Heard with inflammation of pleura; can disappear if sufficient pleural fluid accumulates

   Differentiate pleural from pericardial friction rub: have the patient hold his breath for a few seconds; a rub that persists without respiratory movement must be pericardial; a sound that disappears during apnea and reappears with breathing must be pleural

PALPATION FOR TACTILE VOCAL FREMITUS

Goal. Confirm suspected impaired air transmission (see Auscultatory Percussion).

Technique.

1. Appose the side of your hand or the DIP joints (Fig. 7.7) to a portion of the patient's chest.
2. Ask the patient to repeatedly vocalize "99."

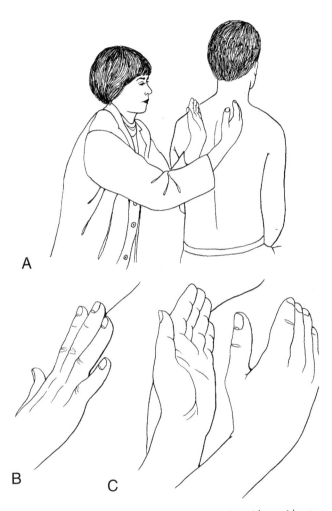

Figure 7.7 Fremitus is best assessed by comparing side to side at a given level. **A.** This examiner uses the sides of both hands. **B.** This technique, better still, employs the metacarpophalangeal joints and sequential testing. **C.** Here the sides are checked simultaneously. Any combination of sensor and timing can be productive except use of the fingertips, which are poor vibratory sensors.

3. Compare the symmetric points on the two hemithoraces for symmetry of vibration as the hand is moved from apex to base.

Interpretation.

1. Decreased fremitus is found with barriers to transmission of sound, i.e., intrapleural fluid, air, or scarring.
2. Increased fremitus suggests consolidation of lung tissue.

FORCED EXPIRATORY TIME

Goal. Assess the adequacy of expiratory airflow.

Technique. Tell the patient to take a long, slow breath in and hold it, and on signal, force the air out, hard and fast, through his open mouth. Auscultate over the trachea anteriorly, timing the expiration with a watch until the last expiratory noise ceases.

Interpretation. A forced expiration of >6 seconds indicates severe obstructive airway disease.

POSTTUSSIVE/POST-DEEP-BREATHING AUSCULTATION

Goal. Differentiate transient medium-sized airway closure from pathologic airway or alveolar disease.

Technique. Have the patient take two or three deep breaths or cough. Reauscultate an area where crackles or rhonchi were heard before this maneuver.

Interpretation. Resolution of abnormal sounds indicates relief of transient atelectasis or movement of secretions.

AUSCULTATORY PERCUSSION

Goal. Assess for deep (>5 cm below chest wall surface) lung lesions.

Technique.

1. Repetitively tap lightly on the manubrium sterni with your plexor alone.
2. With each tap, assess the sound transmitted through the chest and lung to the diaphragm of the stetho-

scope, which is held at symmetric points along each hemithorax posteriorly.

Interpretation. Asymmetry of sound transmission, as in tactile vocal fremitus, is the clue to deep pathology.

PECTORILOQUY

Goal. Confirm the presence of consolidation.

Technique. Have the patient whisper "66 whiskies, please" while the stethoscope is applied over the suspicious area.

Interpretation. Whispered sound is normally muffled; if whispered words sound clear and comprehensible, the area is consolidated.

EGOPHONY

Goal. Confirm the presence of consolidation.

Technique. Have the patient say "ee" each time he is touched by the stethoscope, which is applied over the suspicious area.

Interpretation. If "ee" is transmitted to the stethoscope as "ay," the lung beneath is consolidated.

8

Heart and Great Vessels

Examination of the heart and great vessels follows inspection of the breasts and palpation of the axillae. It is conducted with the patient supine. Equipment includes a **quiet** room to maximize auscultatory accuracy, good cross-lighting and a **fully bared patient chest** for inspection and auscultation (Table 8.1), warm room and warm examiner hands for comfortable palpation, and a **stethoscope** with both bell and diaphragm.

INSPECTION

Goal. Determine the presence of normal and abnormal cardiovascular motion.

Technique. Face the patient, whose *trunk* is raised 30° from the horizontal. Look for visible pulsations, retractions, or any chest wall motion related to cyclic cardiac events; systematically evaluate the apex, left lower sternal area, and pulmonic and aortic valve areas.

Interpretation. In a minority of adults, the apical impulse is visible in the fourth or fifth intercostal space (ICS) 5–6 cm to the left of the midsternal line. Obesity, highly developed pectoral muscles, and large pendulous breasts can all obscure the apical cardiac impulse.

PALPATION

Goal. Determine the presence of normal and abnormal cardiovascular motion. At the aortic valve focus [right upper sternal border (RUSB)], listen for a systolic thrill especially carefully when a systolic ejection murmur is present.

Technique. With vibratory receptors of interphalangeal or metacarpophalangeal joints, seek the apical impulse in the fourth or fifth ICS near the midclavicular line. The hand must settle on the chest, without additional downward pressure. Hold still for 20 seconds to "tune in" on precordial impulses. If unsuccessful, ask the patient to roll slightly leftward. Note the location, size, force, and duration of the apical thrust at this point of maximal impulse (PMI).

Then place two fingers of your other hand on the right carotid pulse. Time the carotid pulse through several cardiac cycles. It should follow each apical impulse after a slight delay.

Next place your right palm along the left lower sternal border (LLSB) to feel for heaves or **thrills**. The latter are vibrations caused by turbulence of blood flow, which feel like the purring of a tiny kitten. Palpate the left upper sternal border (LUSB) and the RUSB in the right and left second ICSs.

Interpretation. A *left* parasternal lift indicates *right* ventricular hypertrophy and forceful contraction.

The *apical impulse*, when palpable, is <2.5 cm in diameter and is felt in early systole. Although in the left lateral decubitus position the location of the apical impulse is not a reliable indicator of heart size, the diameter, duration beyond the first third of systole, force, and any associated thrill remain diagnostically helpful.

1. *Impalpable and invisible apical impulses* are common in normal people. Medial displacement of the apical impulse occurs with reduced cardiac output, as in adrenocortical insufficiency, and with compression of the heart by hyperinflated lungs.

2. *Nonapical cardiac impulses* can be misconstrued as medial displacement of the apical beat, particularly if the apical impulse itself is not palpable. A nonvibratory impulse distinct from the apex beat is a parasternal or right ventricular lift, the best bedside sign for right ventricular myocardial hypertrophy.

3. *Lateral displacement* is seen in left ventricular dilation. This may be physiologically adaptive or may be pathologic and associated with decompensation late in hypertensive heart disease, aortic stenosis, etc.

4. *Apparent lateral displacement* cannot be accepted as accurate if the apex beat is palpable only in the left lateral decubitus position. Late pregnancy may

move the apical impulse lateral to the midclavicular line and superior to the fourth ICS. The impulse may be increased in intensity and diameter.

5. *Left ventricular hypertrophy* does not displace the PMI despite its increasing in force, duration, and size. An isolated increase in force may also reflect a hyperdynamic circulation. Any *enlarged apical impulse* (>3 cm across) raises the question of dyskinesia.

Thrills are palpable murmurs. It is common to hear a murmur without feeling a thrill. In grading systolic murmurs, a thrill defines grade 4 or above. There are four settings, one at each valve projection site, in which the discovery of a thrill has greatest clinical utility:

1. With a systolic ejection murmur maximal at the RUSB, a corresponding thrill proves that the murmur is aortic stenosis.
2. With a systolic ejection murmur associated with unexplained features presumed to reflect *right*-heart strain, a thrill at the second left ICS demonstrates pulmonic stenosis.
3. With a holosystolic murmur that appears equal at the LLSB and the apex, a parasternal thrill excludes mitral regurgitation, while an apical thrill establishes mitral regurgitation.
4. With an apical systolic murmur that is not holosystolic, an apical thrill proves mitral regurgitation.

AUSCULTATION

Goals. Establish a database about cardiovascular function; seek any of multiple abnormalities that produce altered function and characteristic auscultatory findings or constellations.

Technique. Cheap **stethoscopes** often have poor acoustic properties, so expend the money to buy a good one. Beyond instrumentation and knowledge, accurate auscultation of the heart requires system and concentration. For definitions, see Table 8.2.

Listen at five primary sites (Fig. 8.1, *A* and *B*).

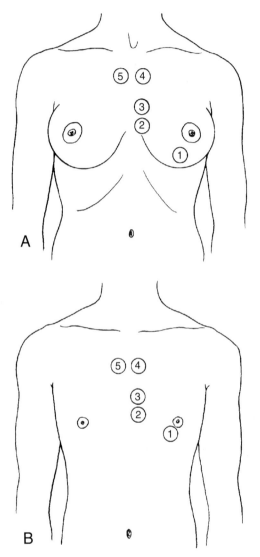

Figure 8.1 Auscultatory sites in women (A) and men (B): *1*, apex; *2*, fourth left ICS (LLSB); *3*, third left ICS; *4*, second left ICS; and *5*, second right ICS.

1. *Apex or mitral:* best located by palpation of the apical beat. If that is impalpable, listen at the left fifth ICS in the midclavicular line. Determine rate and rhythm with the diaphragm held here: Count the apical cardiac rate. (This may exceed the radial pulse rate, chiefly in atrial fibrillation in which it becomes the basis for a pulse deficit [see Chapter 2]). If an irregularity is noted, does it vary with the respiratory cycle?

2. *Left lower sternal border (LLSB),* the tricuspid focus: the fourth ICS just left of the sternal border.

3. *Third left intercostal,* the "accessory pulmonic focus": the third ICS just left of the sternal border.

4. *Second left intercostal,* the LUSB or pulmonic valve focus: the second ICS just left of sternal border.

5. *Second right intercostal,* the aortic valve focus: the second ICS just right of the sternal border (RUSB). Auscultate each area first with the **diaphragm**; repeat with the **bell** held lightly to the skin to listen for lower frequency sounds. At each site, isolate and concentrate on each event in the cycle and listen through enough cycles to characterize all sounds.

Avoid the following common **errors**: Don't listen in a noisy room—the open door lets in noise and destroys privacy; close the door, politely ask the visitors to leave or be silent, and turn off the television. Privacy and modesty need to be respected, but failure to disrobe attenuates all cardiovascular and respiratory vibrations both for palpation and for auscultation and renders both inspection and percussion meaningless. It can also produce sound that is easily misinterpreted as cardiac, not to mention that a shivering patient is miserable (Table 8.1).

Interpretation of rate and rhythm. The normal adult heart beats at 50–100 regular cycles/minute in *normal sinus rhythm.* The athlete's heart may beat slower in *sinus bradycardia,* and slower rates are also found in some heart diseases (Table 2.6). Anemia, hyperthyroidism, fever, or anxiety may push the rate over 100, producing *sinus tachycardia,* even in adults with intrinsically normal cardiovascular sys-

Table 8.1
Adverse Effects of Examination Through Clothing

Obscures genuine diagnostic sound
Creates artifactual sound that is misconstrued as meaningful
May leave patient wondering why the clinician is diffident about
  performing the task (?self-confidence, ?competence)
May make patient wonder why his body is so distasteful as to be
  avoided or examined only cursorily

---

tems, although sinus tachycardia is also common in heart disease.

Sinus arrhythmia is a physiologic irregularity in which the heart rate momentarily increases detectably with inspiration. *Premature contractions* (ventricular or atrial) commonly occur in normal hearts. These produce "extra" or "skipped" beats, without breaking the underlying regularity.

S_1 or First Heart Sound

Technique. Listen early in systole, when ventricular pressure exceeds atrial pressure and the atrioventricular valves close. Determine the presence and consistency of intensity of S_1 **(first heart sound)** from cycle to cycle, then the relative intensity of S_1 at each site. Determine whether S_1 is single or split (Fig. 8.2). If it is split, is the split heard only at the LLSB? If the bell is pressed firmly, the skin functions as a diaphragm, so that transmission of high-pitched sounds suddenly predominates, and this can be capitalized on in distinguishing S_4 (fourth heart sound) from split S_1.

Interpretation. S_1 should be louder at the apex than at the base and should be louder than S_2 (second heart sound) at the apex and softer than S_2 at the base.

Absence of S_1 usually occurs with holosystolic murmurs that have obliterated the sound. *Variable intensity of S_1,* usually coupled with irregularity of rhythm, shows variable atrial filling, usually from atrial fibrillation but sometimes from ventricular arrhythmias.

To determine whether a *"double S_1"* represents S_4 or split S_1, take advantage of the differential pitch (S_1 high, S_4 low) and differential filtering: S_1 is well heard with the diaphragm; S_4 is far better (and often exclusively) heard

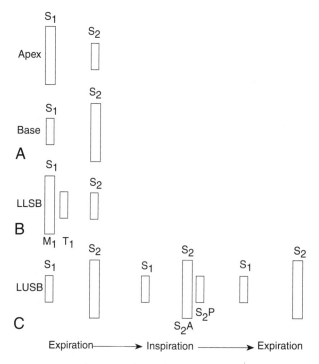

Figure 8.2 Normal variants of S_1 and S_2. **A.** Intensity variations by auscultatory site. **B.** LLSB split of S_1. **C.** Physiologic splitting of S_2.

with the bell held lightly to the skin. With pressure on the bell, S_4 is damped or obliterated, whereas S_1 is unchanged or intensified. Split S_1 sounds are usually best appreciated at LLSB, whereas S_4 sounds of left heart origin are clearest at the apex.

Because of minor asynchrony between left and right ventricular contractions, S_1 may be split at the LLSB, with the loud mitral closure occurring slightly before the softer tricuspid closure.

An *unduly loud S_1* is the earliest physical sign of mitral stenosis and easily recognized when S_1 is louder than S_2 at the second ICS. Loud S_1 sounds are also heard in tachycardia, with short PR intervals, and in hyperkinetic states such as anemia and thyrotoxicosis.

S_2 or Second Heart Sound

Technique. Listen late in systole. As you inch the stethoscope toward the base of the heart, **S_2 (second heart sound)** becomes louder than S_1 at the upper sternal borders. Determine whether S_2 is present and, if it is, what its intensity is relative to S_1.

Then note whether it is single. *Normal physiologic **splitting of S_2*** is exaggerated during inspiration such that the split widens and becomes audible as the patient breathes in, whereas it narrows or disappears as the patient breathes out (Fig. 8.2). This split is best appreciated in the second (or third or, occasionally, fourth) left ICS and is not normally audible at the apex. A split in expiration only is *paradoxical splitting.*

If S_2 is physiologically split, determine the relative intensity of the first component (S_2A, aortic component) compared with the normally softer second component (S_2P, pulmonic component). In normal adults over age 25, S_2A should be much louder.

Interpretation. *"Loud S_2."* Loud S_2 not otherwise qualified refers to a loud aortic component, often with a crisper, higher pitched "tambouric" quality. The most common cause is systemic arterial hypertension.

Soft S_2. All heart sounds grow softer with depression of myocardial function. The differential diagnosis of global heart sound attenuation also includes pericardial effusion, pneumothorax, and emphysema. Such mechanisms, however, do not selectively diminish one cardiac sound in relation to another. A soft aortic component of S_2 is described in aortic valvular stenosis but occurs only in a minority of aortic stenoses in the aged. It is insensitive and nonspecific in the aged, in contrast to its significance in younger persons.

Loud S_2P. Above age 25, an S_2P sound that is louder than S_2A sound is abnormal. *But beware:* When splitting is paradoxical, S_2P will precede S_2A, and splitting will occur only in expiration. If you ignore the respiratory phase in which the sound is heard, you may misinterpret S_2A, because it comes last, as an abnormally increased S_2P.

Audible expiratory splitting of S_2. Many normal young people have a narrowly split S_2 in expiration that splits further with inspiration. Having such persons move to the seated position obliterates expiratory splitting. If S_2A and S_2P are individually normal and if the splitting is neither paradoxical nor fixed, the finding is normal. A right bundle-branch block is another common cause.

Paradoxical splitting of S_2. If there is audible expiratory splitting of S_2 but the components of the second sound fuse on inspiration, paradoxical splitting is present. A short differential diagnosis applies: *(a)* delayed electrical activation of the left ventricle, *(b)* delayed mechanical contraction of the left ventricle, or *(c)* premature contraction of the right ventricle. Bear in mind that the sequence of components is reversed: You hear a soft component first, then a loud one (S_2P, then S_2A). Some settings are

1. *Delayed electrical activation* of the left ventricle is seen in left bundle-branch block.
2. *Artificial pacemakers* mimic left bundle-branch block on auscultation.
3. *Delayed mechanical contraction* of the left ventricle can occur with marked myocardial hypertrophy.
4. *Ischemic myocardium* can sometimes display delayed electromechanical coupling, with paradoxical splitting of S_2, with or without left bundle-branch block.

Fixed splitting of S_2. Fixed splitting is continuous static splitting without respiratory variation. Although the classical cause is atrial septal defect,

1. Some cases of atrial septal defect lack this finding.
2. Persistence of the finding after successful surgical closure of atrial septal defects has been reported.
3. This finding rarely occurs in other conditions, including pulmonary embolism.

Systole

Technique. Assess the period of each cycle after S_1 and before S_2. Determine whether it is silent apart from S_1 and S_2. Listen for murmurs (see below), clicks, and prosthetic valve sounds. **Pericardial rubs** and mediastinal crunches may be detected during systole, especially with the patient seated upright. Pericardial rubs have up to three components that encompass portions of both systole and diastole. They are of medium pitch and often sharply localized. They are best heard with the diaphragm and with the patient seated and leaning forward. Pericardial rubs can be evanescent and recurrent.

The techniques regarding **clicks** are
1. Listen for them as discrete sounds separate from and usually crisper than S_1 and S_2.
2. If one is detected, see whether it can be moved "backward" toward S_1 by having the patient stand or perform the Valsalva maneuver.

Interpretation. Pericardial rubs are most characteristic of pericarditis. Mediastinal crunches have been described in pneumomediastinum, in mediastinitis, and in a small subset of left pneumothoraces.

Ejection clicks usually occur early in systole. They are found in aortic and pulmonic stenosis. Ejection clicks are sharp, high-pitched sounds, and their chief importance is *(a)* to be recognized as related to the valvular lesion and not taken for some other sound and *(b)* to be distinguished, if possible, from the mid- to late-systolic nonejection clicks of mitral prolapse. The nonejection click or clicks of mitral prolapse characteristically follow S_1 and precede the murmur of prolapse if a prolapse murmur is present.

Diastole

Technique. Assess the time following S_2 and preceding the next S_1. Determine whether it is silent. If it is not, discriminate by using the bell at the apex whether discrete low-pitched sounds are heard just after S_2 [likely to be S_3 or third heart sound (Fig. 8.3)] or just before S_1 [likely to be S_4 (Fig. 8.3)]. Longer continuous sounds will be murmurs.

If suspicion of a gallop is substantial but one is not heard conventionally, repeat bell auscultation at the apex with the patient in a modified left lateral decubitus position, since low-pitched diastolic sounds (S_4, S_3, and rumbling murmurs of mitral stenosis) may become audible only in this way.

Opening snaps (OS) occur at the apex, at the LLSB, or in between. To find one, inch the diaphragm from the second left ICS downward and then laterally. If it is still not heard, check for a snap during and after having the patient roll into the left lateral decubitus position.

Interpretation. Diastole is usually silent.

S_3 or third heart sound. **S_3 (third heart sound)** is a low-pitched sound occurring 0.12–0.18 seconds after S_2. It occurs in many normal children and healthy young adults but is always abnormal over age 40. It is seen in some cases of mitral regurgitation in the absence of heart failure but oth-

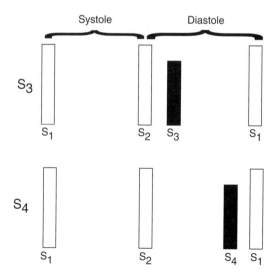

Figure 8.3 Timing of S_3 and S_4 in cardiac cycle.

erwise signifies cardiac failure. The sign is lacking in many patients with proven heart failure, so no inference can be drawn from its absence. Factors that often prevent detection of S_3 include ambient noise, obesity, emphysema, failure to apply the bell precisely to the cardiac apex, excess pressure with the bell, and examination of the seated patient. When S_3 is a critical issue, repeat auscultation with the patient supine and rolled into the left lateral decubitus position.

Right ventricular S_3s are located at the LLSB and often increase with inspiration. A right-heart gallop may radiate to the right supraclavicular fossa; left-heart gallops do not.

S_4 or fourth heart sound. **S_4 (fourth heart sound)** is a low-pitched atrial contraction sound occurring in late diastole. It is often heard in persons over age 50 without evidence of cardiac disease but, when heard in patients under age 50, suggests noncompliance of the ventricle (usually the left). It cannot be present in atrial fibrillation, since it reflects coordinated atrial contraction.

Right atrial gallops may produce S_4 sounds best heard at LLSB. See above for its distinction from a split S_1.

If the heart rate is over 100 beats/minute, discrimination of S_3s from S_4s is impossible, and a "galloping" triple rhythm is designated as a **summation gallop** (unless there is atrial fibrillation, which precludes S_4).

Opening snaps (OS) are sharp diastolic sounds that are best known in mitral stenosis. They are of medium to high pitch and sometimes tightly localized. When an opening snap occurs rapidly after S_2, the mitral stenosis is severe. OS can disappear in mitral stenosis, however, when valve leaflets have become heavily calcified. OS can mimic S_3.

Heart Murmurs

Technique. Rudiments of murmur description are given in Table 8.2. Listen in both systole and diastole for any long vibrations that occupy a quarter of the phase or more and are not so sharp and distinct as the preceding sounds. If they are found, characterize them by loudness, locale of greatest intensity, shape (configuration), pitch (frequency), duration of radiation, and response to maneuvers (below).

Table 8.2
Murmurs: Definition of Descriptive Terms

Loudness (intensity) of systolic murmurs
  Grade 1: barely audible with careful concentration
  Grade 2: faint but readily detected
  Grade 3: prominent, easily detectable
  Grade 4: louder still; palpable thrill associated
  Grade 5: audible with only rim of stethoscope touching chest wall
  Grade 6: loud enough to be heard without stethoscope

Shape (configuration)
  Crescendo: rising in intensity

  Crescendo-decrescendo (diamond-shaped): rising, then falling in
    intensity

  Box-shaped: even in intensity

Timing and duration in cycle
  Duration or relationship to S_1 and S_2, including obliteration of
    either or both of them

Interpretation. *Innocent murmurs.* There are many **innocent murmurs,** including some in children, adults, pregnant and lactating women, and the aged. Characteristics that are aggregately associated with innocence are

- Absence of cardiorespiratory symptoms with exercise
- Normal, regular apical pulse rate and respiratory rate
- Normal carotid upstrokes, jugular venous pressure, and jugular waveforms
- Normal lung examination
- Normal location and character of apex beat
- Absence of associated thrill
- Normal timing and characteristics of S_1 and S_2
- Absence of associated diastolic murmur
- Short duration, occupying one-half of systole or less
- Absence of S_3 if patient is over age 40
- Absence of second systolic murmur elsewhere in the precordium
- Absence of augmentation by Valsalva maneuver
- If extant, normal chest x-ray, electrocardiogram, and echocardiogram

Many patients with systolic ejection murmurs fail some of these criteria but lack heart disease. Conversely, serious pathology may slip through this imperfect net, e.g., hypertrophic cardiomyopathy in an asymptomatic young athlete whose murmur does not increase with the Valsalva maneuver.

Mitral prolapse. Consider a diagnosis of **mitral prolapse** with the following findings:

- If S_1 is followed by a midsystolic click and a "square" murmur occupies systole beyond this point, mitral prolapse is present and includes some valvular regurgitation.
- If there is no murmur but there is one or more mid- or late-systolic click(s) best heard at the apex, mitral prolapse is probable.
- Murmurs that obliterate both S_1 and S_2 at the apex are less likely to be mitral prolapse and are more likely to be nonprolapse mitral regurgitation.
- Mitral prolapse can change auscultatory features from day to day. A more prominent mitral regurgitation

murmur on a second visit does not necessarily mean that a case of mitral prolapse is progressing.

Holosystolic murmurs. The chief **holosystolic murmurs** are mitral regurgitation and tricuspid regurgitation. *Tricuspid regurgitation* should be louder at the LLSB than at the apex, but *mitral regurgitation* is the reverse. Radiation to the axilla is far more typical of mitral regurgitation. Radiation to the epigastrium slightly favors tricuspid regurgitation. Associated signs are also of help: Giant v waves or pulsatile hepatomegaly proves tricuspid regurgitation, but these high-specificity signs are uncommon.

Diastolic murmurs. **Diastolic murmurs** almost always signify structural heart disease. They are graded 1–4. The commonest diastolic murmur, *aortic insufficiency*, begins with or just after S_2A and tails off in diastole. The peripheral signs of aortic insufficiency are discredited. In seeking this murmur, you must constantly "reset" the ears and brain to listen for a high-pitched sound that is closer in frequency to breath sounds than to other murmurs.

Pulmonic insufficiency, the Graham Steell murmur, should be loudest at the right sternal border but overlaps aortic insufficiency. Pulmonary hypertension, marked by an accentuated S_2P, makes pulmonic insufficiency more likely.

Mitral stenosis produces a rumbling murmur that is best heard in early diastole and during atrial systole and is loudest at the apex or medial to it. Having the patient roll into the left lateral decubitus position can enhance the audibility of this murmur.

Aged patients with basal systolic murmurs. Valvular heart disease increases in the elderly, but so do innocuous murmurs. Pathologic conditions may produce deceptively minimal physical signs. The commonest troublesome evaluation is of a grade 2 systolic ejection murmur, maximal at the RUSB, without radiation to the neck, alteration in the carotid upstrokes, reduction of S_2A, lowering of either the systolic blood pressure or the pulse pressure, or the harshness found in some aortic stenoses. In the aged with aortic stenosis, in contrast to younger patients with the same valve lesion,

- The murmur is frequently softer and shorter.
- The murmur may not radiate to the neck.
- The carotid upstroke is seldom attenuated or delayed.
- S_2A often appears falsely normal.
- The systolic blood pressure may be normal or even high.
- The pulse pressure need not be decreased even by severe aortic stenosis.

Aortic stenosis and insufficiency separately and together. When you detect aortic stenosis, check for aortic insufficiency. In a patient with aortic insufficiency, some basal systolic murmurs relate exclusively to high blood flow across a valve with normal forward flow characteristics.

The *Gallavardin phenomenon* is an acoustic alteration whereby aortic stenosis becomes louder and more musical at the apex. Think of it when you are tempted to diagnose multiple different systolic murmurs in a single person.

MANIPULATIONS OF MURMURS AND HEART SOUNDS

Overall goal. Correctly infer the locale and nature of abnormal sounds that have been detected.

Locale and Transmission

Technique. Murmurs are usually loudest where they arise; thus, close attention to this and to recording it often suffices to characterize the murmur satisfactorily. When confused, consider the following:

1. Forward flow from the aortic valve is loudest in the RUSB.
2. Aortic insufficiency may be loudest over the sternum or at either sternal edge, halfway down, or over a clavicle.
3. Sound best heard at the LUSB should arise from forward flow across the pulmonic valve.
4. The LLSB reflects right ventricular and tricuspid valvular events.
5. The apex is the prime mitral acoustic area.

Interpretation. Many murmurs propagate in attenuated form from the point of origin. Certain characteristic murmur radiations are *(a)* mitral murmurs to the axillae, *(b)* aortic forward flow murmurs to the carotids, and *(c)* some pulmonic murmurs to the interscapular area (high specificity, low sensitivity).

Body Position Maneuvers

Technique. Listen with the patient in various positions, e.g., left lateral decubitus, seated, squatting, abruptly arising from a squat. Rollover of the patient from the supine to the left lateral decubitus position increases the audibility of gallops and some murmurs. Place the bell of the stethoscope on the apex with the patient supine, and listen as the patient turns. With the stethoscope head held lightly on the apex, say, "Now while I listen, when I say so, roll halfway over onto your left side, away from me." Listen during the transfer—and for a few seconds afterward.

Interpretation. The left lateral decubitus position enhances gallops and can bring out the opening snap and the murmur of mitral stenosis. Left lateral decubitus positioning can bring out an S_3 or S_4 that was previously occult.

Rapid standing abruptly reduces venous return. Murmurs of mitral prolapse and hypertrophic cardiomyopathy are often loudened.

Squatting has unpredictable effects on systolic murmurs including mitral regurgitation other than prolapse. It increases most aortic insufficiency murmurs and brings out some that were silent before.

Sitting may disclose pericardial rubs and aortic insufficiency murmurs not heard before. The legs may be dangled. When the position is chosen because of suspected aortic insufficiency, leaning forward is also included.

Valsalva Maneuver

Technique. Tell the patient to push out the abdomen as far as possible, with a sustained effort. There should be no air movement, the patient's face should turn red, and the patient's veins should pop up some seconds after the maneuver has been in progress. Ask the patient to push this way while you listen uninterruptedly. End by saying,

"Breathe normally," after 15 seconds. Continue auscultation for another 15 seconds, attending to murmur intensity or timing of events, with comparison to baseline at several distinct points in time: *(a)* 5–10 seconds after initiation, *(b)* immediately on release, *(c)* 1–2 heartbeats after release, and *(d)* 4–6 heartbeats after release.

Interpretation. Many patients cannot perform a Valsalva maneuver. Others make so much noncardiac noise that cardiac sound becomes indistinguishable. If cardiac sound is assessable, most murmurs decrease during the strain phase, but two-thirds of hypertrophic cardiomyopathy murmurs increase. However, there is a disturbing 30% rate of unexplained murmur *reduction* in hypertrophic cardiomyopathy.

On release of strain, resumption of normal murmur intensity within 1 or 2 heartbeats suggests right-heart origin. A delay for several additional beats implicates the left heart.

Handgrip Test

Technique. Sustained handgrip increases heart rate and blood pressure. Tell the patient, "While I listen, please grip this ball (or my fingers) as hard as you can. *Don't stop breathing.* Keep up the tight squeezing until I tell you to stop, and remember to breathe normally." This maneuver is contraindicated in symptomatic unstable coronary artery disease (unstable angina pectoris or acute myocardial infarction) and symptomatic aortic stenosis and, if chest pain or breathlessness results in any patient, is stopped at once.

Interpretation. When feasible and safe, sustained handgrip increases murmur intensity in two-thirds of patients with mitral regurgitation or ventricular septal defect, in a minority of patients with aortic stenosis (on whom you should not perform this test!), and in fewer patients with right-heart murmurs. It decreases the murmur of hypertrophic cardiomyopathy very consistently but, "paradoxically," also reduces some mitral regurgitation murmurs. This test does not display sufficiently distinct patterns to permit systolic murmur diagnosis but can bring out an S_3 or S_4 that was previously occult.

Passive Straight-Leg Raising Maneuver

Technique. With passive straight-leg raising, right-heart return increases almost at once, and left-heart return increases soon afterward. Have an assistant raise both the patient's legs and thighs to 75° of hip flexion. During continued auscultation, note the immediate effect on cardiac sound and any effect that is delayed 4–6 heartbeats, as well as changes immediately after and 4–6 heartbeats after the legs and thighs are relowered.

Interpretation. Passive straight-leg raising mimics some effects of squatting, thus making many murmurs increase. Most murmurs due to hypertrophic cardiomyopathy are reduced, however.

In deciding about chamber of origin, if passive straight-leg raising causes an S_3 to appear 4 or 5 heartbeats after the maneuver is undertaken and the gallop persists 4 or 5 heartbeats after release, left ventricular origin is more likely. If responses occur within the first or second heartbeat, right ventricular origin is probable.

Aortic Insufficiency Maneuvers

Technique. Listen with the diaphragm. Tune in for a very high- pitched diastolic sound after S_2.

1. Have the seated patient lean forward as far as possible, exhale deeply, and cease breathing for a few seconds.
2. Or have the patient assume a knee-chest or knee-elbow (dog) position on the bed, so that the heart settles toward the anterior chest wall.
3. Or have the patient lie prone (face down) on the bed. Then have the patient turn his head away while you slip the diaphragm of the stethoscope between the sternum and the mattress or between the patient's breasts, with or without breath-holding in expiration.

Interpretation. A high-pitched diastolic murmur brought out or loudened by any of these maneuvers is likely to be aortic valvular insufficiency. If it is loudest down the left sternal border, it is probably from the valve proper; if it is loudest down the right sternal border, it is probably from the supravalvular ring of the ascending aorta.

Cycled Respiration Test

Technique. The intentionally slow, deep breathing of cycled respiration gives you an opportunity to observe the effects of inspiration and expiration on heart sounds and murmurs. Remind the patient to breathe through the nose for this maneuver. (Oral breathing enhances airway sound.) Several breathing cycles are auscultated. Many patients perform a Valsalva maneuver when asked to hold the breath, so a better request is, "Please stop breathing for a moment."

Breath-holding itself helps discriminate pericardial from pleural rubs but has no role in determining the splitting of S_2.

Interpretation. Cardiac sound that softens on inspiration and loudens on expiration usually comes from the left heart, and cardiac sound that increases with inspiration usually comes from the right side of the heart. The only common exceptions are patients with marked air trapping in whom all cardiac sound diminishes in concert on inspiration and patients with pulmonic stenosis murmurs that soften on inspiration.

Inspiratory augmentation is highly characteristic of tricuspid regurgitation. Many left-sided systolic murmurs do not change with the respiratory phase. Those that do, diminish on inspiration and increase on expiration.

If tricuspid regurgitation is suspected and inspiratory augmentation of a holosystolic murmur *(Carvallo's sign)* has been negative, the abdominojugular test is performed. If there is no change with the abdominojugular test, both tests are done together, constituting *Gooch's test*. If the murmur increases, tricuspid regurgitation is very likely.

Transient Arterial Occlusion Maneuver

Technique. Measure the systolic blood pressure. Then have an assistant place a sphygmomanometer around each upper arm of the patient and inflate both cuffs 30 torr above the systolic pressure. Any change in cardiac sound over the

ensuing 30 seconds is noted, as are any changes for the 30
seconds after deflating both cuffs.

Interpretation. At 20 seconds after transient arterial
occlusion, many mitral regurgitation and ventricular septal
defect murmurs increase; none decrease. Other systolic
murmurs remain constant or decrease. The maneuver does
not discriminate between mitral regurgitation and ventricular septal defect.

Amyl Nitrite Test

Technique. When administering the amyl nitrite test,
advise the patient that "any nausea, light-headedness, or
racing pulse will last only briefly." Have the patient lie
down to avoid fainting, and begin auscultation. Have an
assistant measure the patient's blood pressure and leave the
cuff in place. The ampule of amyl nitrite is broken, and the
patient inhales the drug. The expended ampule is dropped
into a cup of water. The patient's blood pressure should
decline sharply within 30 seconds, with reflex increase in
heart rate. Amyl nitrite is contraindicated in pregnancy,
with hypertension, and with severe aortic stenosis.

Interpretation. Murmurs of left-sided regurgitant
lesions—aortic insufficiency and mitral regurgitation—tend
to decrease with amyl nitrite inhalation. Innocuous aortic
flow murmurs, aortic stenosis murmurs, and hypertrophic
cardiomyopathy murmurs usually increase. Tricuspid
regurgitation and mitral stenosis increase also.

If the issue is a forward flow murmur from the left ventricular outflow tract versus mitral regurgitation, discrimination is good.

In diastolic murmur characterization, pulmonic insufficiency increases or remains constant, in contrast to diminution of aortic insufficiency.

Abdominojugular Maneuver for Murmurs

Technique. To use the abdominojugular maneuver to
test for murmurs, have the patient lie supine and breathe
normally. Apply pressure to the patient's midabdomen to
illustrate what will be done. Counsel against an inadvertent

Valsalva maneuver or other breath-holding. Auscultate and press with your palm and slightly spread fingers. Keep up the pressure for 10 seconds at about 20 mm Hg. Auscultate during compression and for 10 seconds afterward.

If no conclusion is possible from the cycled respiration test or with the abdominojugular maneuver alone, the two manipulations are combined. Have the patient, after full exhalation, take an unusually deep and slow inspiration for as long as possible, short of breath-holding, while you press the patient's abdomen as before. Continue auscultation after sudden release of both inspired air and abdominal pressure; sharp *reduction* in sound may be more acoustically recognizable than slow augmentation.

Interpretation. Augmentation of holosystolic murmur intensity with deep inspiration and/or with abdominal pressure strongly suggests tricuspid rather than mitral regurgitation.

INSPECTION, PALPATION AND AUSCULTATION OF GREAT ARTERIES

Goal. Determine characteristics of cardiac outflow and the intrinsic character of carotid arterial flow.

Technique. Palpate each side of the patient's neck separately, inferior to the mandibular ramus and lateral to the trachea, for the carotid artery pulse. Its upstroke coincides with the midpoint of ventricular systole. If you auscultate the heart while feeling the carotid, the carotid pulse will accompany S_1 or follow shortly after it. You can palpate the carotids sequentially—never simultaneously—giving attention to the variable force of the pulse from side to side.

With the patient's face turned very slightly toward the opposite side, gently press the bell as high on the carotid artery as possible. Systolic sounds are usually audible, corresponding to transmission of S_2 and sometimes of S_1. The intensity of transmitted sound should be symmetrical. Listen for murmurs in the neck.

Don't listen too low in the neck or too far anteriorly or posteriorly. All these errors can obscure sounds of interest and may introduce insignificant and confusing sound. Don't apply excess pressure to the artery, which can produce arterial obstruction and stroke: Gentleness remains the watchword, whether palpating with digits or touching with the head of the stethoscope. A lesser degree of excess pressure on the carotid can create artifactual systolic sound.

Interpretation. On inspection, a visible and palpable arterial pulsation resulting from tortuosity of the aortic arch is often detected in the supraclavicular area or in the suprasternal (jugular) notch.

The right and left carotid pulsations should be equal in amplitude and should have a single positive wave. If they are unequal, aortic outflow tract disease cannot be invoked to explain the decreased side. Differential signs from side to side implicate lesions distal to the common proximal pathway shared by the two vessels.

Global attenuation of pulses raises the prospect of widespread vasculopathy or narrow pulse pressure. The latter can be readily tested by measuring the blood pressure.

A wide pulse pressure can be responsible for increased carotid pulse intensity. Aortic insufficiency or any high cardiac output state can also produce bounding pulses such as are seen in hyperthyroidism, anemia, pregnancy, extreme anxiety, etc.

Carotid Murmurs

Technique.

1. Listen at the right second ICS. If a systolic murmur is heard, inch the stethoscope slowly up, noting whether the sound steadily muffles, peaks in the supraclavicular fossa, or softens above the sternum and then grows louder as you reach the carotid bifurcation.

2. If there is no cardiac murmur or if there is a more prominent sound in the supraclavicular fossa, reauscultate each carotid with the patient's shoulders hyperextended, and note whether the murmur is reduced by this maneuver.

3. If substantial suspicion of a carotid origin persists, palpate the carotid a little longer, trying to ascertain the presence of a palpable systolic arterial shudder.
4. Continuous (systolic-diastolic) murmurs heard over the carotid are presumed to be arterial bruits or cervical venous hums. Listen with the patient upright, and seek obliteration of sound with gentle compression of the jugular outflow at the clavicle.

Interpretation. If there is no systolic murmur at the RUSB, infer that the sound arises from arteries and not from the heart. Some sounds come from the subclavian artery and have no adverse implications; they tend to be obliterated with hyperextension of the shoulders.

In children and young adults, cervical venous hums are common, and carotid arterial bruits are rare. The venous hum is often continuous and louder in diastole, whereas most carotid bruits are exclusively systolic. Carotid bruits are augmented or unchanged when the patient is recumbent; venous hums are reduced or absent when the patient is supine. Light pressure on the jugular outflow just above the clavicle obliterates a venous hum but not a carotid bruit.

If there *is* a basal cardiac murmur, the heart must be considered as a source. Progressive attenuation from the second right interspace to the supraclavicular fossa to the carotid bifurcation is characteristic of an aortic valvular murmur with propagation. Coexistent valvular and arterial lesions can produce loud sound at the RUSB, a falloff in the supraclavicular fossa, and resumption of loudness over the carotid bifurcation.

If vibrations are palpable in the carotid, constituting a shudder, the source can be arterial or a transmitted aortic stenosis.

If partial release of pressure on the stethoscope causes the carotid murmur to disappear, the murmur may be an artifact of iatrogenic turbulence via excess pressure—and never repeat the mistake, which can be hazardous as well as misleading.

GREAT VEIN ASSESSMENT

Goals. Determine central venous pressure and the state of the right heart and assess intravascular fluid status.

Technique. Observe the lateral neck for visibility of the jugular venous blood column and its height. With a light beam directed tangential to the right side of the neck, observe for pulsations. Inspect the right external jugular vein for outward wave components. Test for vein patency by gentle compression of the jugular outflow against the clavicle, which should bring up the visibility of the blood column. Observe during inspiration; progressively lower the head of the bed and, with it, the patient's trunk until the veins come into view. Neck vein inspection is aided by relieving tension on the neck muscles, minimizing flexion of the neck on the chest.

Look at the height of the external **jugular venous blood column** and at waveforms in the much less distinct internal jugular. Inspiration normally lowers jugular venous pressure.

If large **jugular pulsations** are observed, time them with respect to audible heart sounds. An outward and/or upward bulge just before S_1 will be an "a" wave from right atrial contraction. Normally, this is the most prominent jugular pulsation. A bulge that coincides with S_2 will be a "v" wave, reflecting right ventricular contraction.

Interpretation. Many persons with fleshy necks have unassessable jugular blood columns.

The normal central venous pressure ranges from 4 to 9 cm of water. The sternal angle lies 5 cm above the midpoint of the right atrium. Thus, in normal persons, the apex of the jugular venous blood column will lie up to 4 cm above the sternal angle. Always keep in mind that *the height of the blood column, not its length, matters* and that 5 is added to the observed height to produce the **estimated central venous pressure**.

A jugular venous pressure corresponding to an estimated central venous pressure over 12 cm of water is highly suggestive of right-heart failure complicated by systemic venous hypertension. When the scenario has inconsistencies, check the opposite jugular and consider the sources of misleading jugular venous pressure elevation.

When one jugular venous pressure substantially exceeds the other, decide which of the two jugular veins is the accurate marker of intrathoracic events. Variability of column height with respiratory cycle, with change in body position, and/or with the abdominojugular maneuver suggests the accurate side; lack of response tends to point to the misleading vessel. *The more normal-looking column height is not always the accurate one.* Consider whether

- There is proximal obstruction of the more distended vein.
- The "flat" vein is nonpatent, therefore not reflective of central venous pressure.
- Abnormal or aberrant venous valves mask or mimic central venous hypertension.
- The patient has idiopathic jugular venous ectasia.

Proximal obstruction will usually be obvious if it is part of a superior vena cava syndrome. An uncoiled atherosclerotic aorta may pinch the termination of either jugular, as may an ectatic atherosclerotic aorta or a dissecting hematoma of the aorta.

The differential diagnosis of *persistently flat external jugular veins* includes venous hypotension, characteristically from marked intravascular volume depletion, and fibrous obliteration of the venous lumen. The Trendelenburg position will usually bring out a blood column in any patent jugular, even with hypovolemia, but cannot open up a solid cord. At times, cautious intravascular volume repletion may assist this assessment. Aged patients may have obliterated veins, as, for other reasons, may intravenous drug abusers and persons with central vascular catheters. Such individuals need not have had clinical jugular thrombophlebitis to develop late scarring and luminal obliteration.

Normally, a single prominent pulsation is seen in the neck with each heartbeat, and that is the carotid pulse. A prominent outward pulsation before the carotid pulse, just before S_1 and synchronous with S_4, if there is one, will be a giant "a" wave representing excessively prominent atrial contraction in *tricuspid stenosis*. These and giant "a" waves in *right ventricular hypertrophy* are *regular* in timing. The appearance of *intermittent* "cannon a waves" suggests that the right atrium is sometimes contracting against a closed tricuspid valve. A prominent outward pulsation after the carotid "c" wave, nearly coincident with S_2A, will be a giant "v" wave. These occur in *tricuspid regurgitation*. Irregular giant "v" waves are sometimes seen in *atrial fibrillation* even without tricuspid regurgitation.

Venous waves are often difficult to distinguish from carotid pulsations. To differentiate the two, recall that

1. The jugular venous pulse can have up to three positive components; the carotid artery pulse has only one.
2. On inspiration, the level of the venous column normally descends; the carotid pulsation remains visible above this point.
3. *Light* pressure over the vein just above the medial clavicle will eliminate a venous pulse but will not affect carotid pulses.

Abdominojugular Test for Veins

Technique. The abdominojugular test described above for murmur manipulation can be applied to venous pressure if there is an assessable jugular venous blood meniscus. The new variable measured is visible *jugular blood column height*. Check the jugular venous column height, then observe the jugular column through 10 seconds of Valsalva-free non-breath-holding firm abdominal compression and for a few seconds after sudden release of this pressure on the abdomen.

Interpretation. If jugular pressure stays steady, the test is normal. If the pressure promptly rises, then drops rapidly back to normal while compression continues, this too is negative. When, however, there is a prompt rise of 4 cm or more that is sustained throughout the 10 seconds, and then a prompt drop of 4 cm or more on release, the result is abnormal and associated with an elevated pulmonary arterial wedge pressure, i.e., *left*-heart dysfunction and increased central blood volume. The test may also be positive in patients with a recent right ventricular myocardial infarction.

Kussmaul's Sign

Technique. Find the top of the jugular blood column. Observe whether the pressure rises or falls on slow inspiration during cycled respiration. The paradoxical elevation of venous pressure with inspiration is called Kussmaul's sign.

Interpretation. When jugular venous pressure rises on inspiration, the differential diagnosis includes pericardial constriction (but not cardiac tamponade), right ventricular myocardial infarction, congestive heart failure, acute cor pulmonale, and restrictive heart disease. One key distinction is between constriction and tamponade, which share many features. Kussmaul's sign will strongly favor the former; its absence, the latter.

9

Abdomen

After completing cardiac examination, move on to examination of the abdomen. The patient is to remain recumbent. A gown is used to cover the patient's chest, and a half-sheet or similar drape is used to cover the patient's groin. You should have warm hands, a warm stethoscope diaphragm, good lighting, and complete exposure of the abdominal wall. Examine from the patient's right side. *Begin the abdominal examination with inspection, followed by auscultation, percussion, and palpation last.*

Vital **surface landmarks** include costal margins, the xiphoid process, and the iliac crests. The highest points of the iliac crests lie at the level of the 4th lumbar vertebra, 2–8 cm caudad to the 12th rib tip. Also key are *(a)* the anterior superior iliac spines and *(b)* the pubic crest and tubercles that define the inferior bony boundaries of the abdomen and pelvis, respectively. The inguinal ligament divides the abdomen from the thigh.

The position of the navel varies with habitus. The abdomen is described by quadrants: right lower and left lower (RLQ and LLQ, respectively) and right upper and left upper (RUQ and LUQ, respectively). Right and left refer to the *patient's* right and left (Fig. 9.1). Key points of visceral anatomy are

- The upper border of the **liver** lies under ribs 7–11 in the RUQ, curves across the midline, and continues to a point near the *left* nipple. The sharp lower liver edge follows the right costal margin and ends over the gastric pylorus.
- The **gallbladder** lies at the lateral border of the rectus abdominis below the costal margin.
- The **pancreas** sits deep in the retroperitoneum behind the stomach in the LUQ. Even when enlarged it is nonpalpable.
- The **stomach** lies deep in the LUQ.

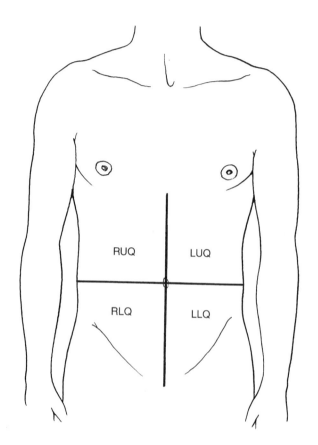

Figure 9.1 Routine abdominal area designations by quadrantic division. *RUQ,* right upper quadrant; *LUQ,* left upper quadrant; *RLQ,* right lower quadrant; *LLQ,* left lower quadrant.

- The **spleen** underlies the left rib cage parallel to ribs 9–11. Unless enlarged to thrice-normal size, it cannot be palpated in adults.
- The **aorta** bifurcates at the level of the navel. It lies immediately anterior to and slightly to the left of the vertebrae.

- The *lower pole* of each **kidney** lies just above the transumbilical plane.
- The **urinary bladder**, if very full, may project out from behind the symphysis pubis and become palpable through the abdominal wall.

INSPECTION

Goal. Seek regional or generalized abdominal disturbance.

Technique. Note contour, movement, and skin. Assess the navel for protuberance. The skin of the abdomen is studied for surgical scars (Fig. 9.2). In thin patients, epigastric or periumbilical transmitted aortic pulsations may be visible. Observe for peristaltic movement and the normally faint rise (with inspiration) and fall of the abdominal wall.

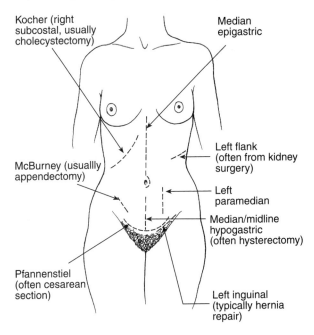

Figure 9.2 Common locations of classic abdominal surgical scars.

Interpretation. The extremes of contour are protuberant distension and the scaphoid or sunken abdomen. A *newly* protuberant navel suggests an increase in intra-abdominal pressure, e.g., from ascites. Evaluation of distension, masses, ascites, organomegaly, and vascular abnormalities is discussed below.

AUSCULTATION

Goal. Determine the presence of normal and abnormal sounds from intestinal motility, vascular flow, and peritoneal respiratory motion.

Technique. With the diaphragm of the stethoscope held to any quadrant, **bowel sounds** are normally readily appreciated as intermittent gurgles.

Interpretation. There is a wide range of normality in abundance of bowel sounds. If none are heard for 1 full minute, infer **ileus** (see below).

PERCUSSION

Goals. Define the positions and size of solid and hollow viscera and assess masses.

Technique. In screening, percussion is used primarily to outline the liver and the resonant, gas-containing hollow viscera that fill the abdomen.

Dullness to percussion distinguishes liver from resonant lung above and from air-containing bowel below. Beginning at the right fourth intercostal space, percuss *caudally* in the right midclavicular line. When resonance of the lung changes to dullness, the upper border of the liver has been reached; mark this level. Percuss *cephalad* from bowel resonance up to the dull inferior border of the liver. Measure the liver span from the upper to the lower border of dullness.

The overfilled **urinary bladder**, when rising above the symphysis pubis, may be percussed as a globular dullness, but as with the spleen, screening bladder percussion is not useful.

Interpretation. Percussion of the liver is an imperfect method. A span exceeding 12 cm at the midclavicular line on the right suggests enlargement.

LIGHT PALPATION

Goal. Assess near-surface structures and tenderness.

Technique. A finger pressed into the umbilical depression will normally meet with fascial resistance, indicating intact underlying fascia. In *diastasis recti*, the recti abdominis have a muscular defect large enough to admit the fingertips, but the subjacent musculofascial layers resist further insertion. Having the patient raise the head from the table brings out diastasis or a ventral hernia.

Light palpation is uncomfortable for the ticklish. Deep palpation using firm, constant pressure is better tolerated.

Interpretation. Innocuous subcutaneous masses such as lipomas are found by light palpation. Ticklishness can be psychologic in origin although involuntary; tenderness is much more often organic.

A liver edge palpable more than 2 cm below the right costal margin, in the absence of pulmonary hyperinflation, suggests hepatomegaly.

REGULAR (DEEPER) PALPATION

Goal. Discover information about the size of the organs and the presence and character of abnormalities, including masses.

Technique. After each quadrant has been lightly palpated, warn the patient that you will be feeling deep in the abdomen, and casually ask that he let you know if you touch a sore spot. If the patient has tensed up during light palpation, have him flex his hips and knees slightly; this facilitates relaxation of abdominal musculature. Begin with a touch just firm enough to overcome skin sensitivity. Use the palmar surface of the approximated fingers of one or both hands, proceeding from quadrant to quadrant. Press downward 1–4 cm. Assess for tenderness, superficial masses, and hyperesthesia and/or dysesthesia.

If abdominal pain is at issue, reserve deep palpation of the area in question until last. Watch the patient's face during palpation: Many persons who do not speak of pain show their discomfort by facial change. Painful palpation often stimulates wide opening of the eyes expressing apprehension.

To feel the *liver edge,*

1. Place apposed fingers deep into the patient's RUQ, 2 cm caudal to the margin previously determined by percussion.
2. Have the patient inhale deeply and exhale slowly, repeatedly if necessary (Fig. 9.3A).
3. The liver edge descends slightly with inspiration and slides over your fingers. It feels solid yet soft.

An alternative method is

1. Curl your fingers from above over the lower rib margin deep into the RUQ.
2. Have the patient breathe deeply and slowly (Fig. 9.3B).

Assess the liver edge, if felt, for consistency, clarity or "sharpness" of margin, contour, and tenderness.

To detect **splenomegaly**, have the patient roll into the right lateral decubitus position. With your left hand pressing into the patient's left flank from behind the lower margin of the rib cage, press your right hand up and back beneath the patient's anterior rib cage. The spleen descends with the diaphragm, so have the patient inhale, then exhale. Assess the organ, if palpable, for consistency, tenderness, and size.

Deep palpation in the midline near the umbilicus may define margins of the aorta in a thin person or a person with a lax abdominal wall. Use both hands; press deeply on either side of the aorta. Estimate width.

Renal palpation is attempted by elevating the flank with your nondominant hand and pressing the dominant hand deep medially and upward under the rib cage.

If dullness is present suprapubically, palpation may reveal a full urinary bladder or an enlarged uterus. Full bladders are sometimes soft and variably compressible.

Inguinofemoral lymph nodes along the inguinal ligament and in the femoral triangle are superficial and, even in normal hosts, are often palpable. They are small, soft, and freely mobile.

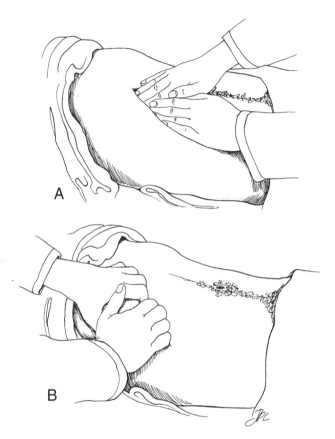

Figure 9.3 *A.* Palpation of liver edge. Press deeply beneath the right costal margin to "flip" the liver edge as it moves upward on expiration if you are unsure whether it has descended to touch your fingers on inspiration. *B.* Alternative "hook" method for assessing an elusive liver margin.

You can examine the femoral arteries during examination of the abdomen. The femoral artery pulsates just above or below the inguinal ligament.

Interpretation. Innocuous findings from regular palpation of the abdomen are numerous (Table 9.1).

Table 9.1
Normal Variants and Common Abnormalities

Inspection	Percussion
Localized or generalized protuberance	Air/gas variants
Fat	Liver span range
Flatus	Urine-filled bladder
Feces	Pregnant uterus
Fetus	
Fluid (ascites)	Palpation
Neoplasms	Diastasis recti and
Local or small contour irregularities	incisional hernias
Cutaneous or subcutaneous tumors	Innocuous subcutaneous
Scars with retraction or puckering	masses
Skin	Colonic feces
Nonpigmented striae	Lower border of liver
Pattern of venous flow	Aortic pulsation
Common benign lesions	Lower pole of right
Hemangiomas	kidney (rare)
Seborrheic keratoses	Urine-filled bladder
Nevi	Pregnant uterus
	Small inguinofemoral
Auscultation	lymph nodes
Range of bowel sounds	
Normal cardiovascular sound	
Transmitted	
Local	

The normal consistency of the abdomen is soft; mobile bowel gives way to deep prodding. The patient may experience discomfort on deep palpation of the epigastrium and of the LLQ, but normally there is *no sharp or localized pain* elicited by this maneuver. Also, unless your hands are cold or you push too rapidly or too deeply, the abdomen does not resist palpation. Except for the commonly palpable, stool-distended descending and sigmoid colons and, rarely, a cecum, bowel segments cannot be distinguished by palpation.

Normal livers are frequently impalpable. The edge of a normal liver will not extend more than 2 cm below the right costal margin. When palpable, the liver margin is distinct, smooth, soft to slightly firm, and minimally tender. See the appropriate section below.

Normal spleens are impalpable in adults. See the appropriate section below.

Normal kidneys are rarely felt. The lower pole of a normal kidney can yield a firm, rounded tip deep in the flank, particularly if the kidney is ptotic.

Palpation and percussion are notoriously insensitive for detection of bladder enlargement.

ABDOMINAL PAIN EVALUATION

Goal. Determine the severity, acuity, locale, and etiopathogenesis of abdominal pain as guides to intervention and prognosis.

Technique. *History.* In addition to usual characterization, think about visceral pain projections (Fig. 9.4, *A* and *B*). From the past medical history, focus on past abdominal pain and prior abdominal surgery. Ask about the following systems:

- *Gastrointestinal:* Nausea, vomiting, hematemesis; diarrhea, constipation, change in stool habits or characteristics, bloody or tarry stools (melena); jaundice, pruritus, dark urine; change in abdominal contour; alcohol and medication history; prior cholecystitis or pancreatitis
- *Genitourinary:* History of renal stone, gout, urinary tract infection or hematuria; flank pain or lower back pain; frequency or hesitancy; menstrual history, possibility of pregnancy, spontaneous or therapeutic abortion; sexual history
- *Vascular:* Chest pain or known coronary artery disease (angina pectoris can present as epigastric pain); known aortic disease, postprandial abdominal pain
- *Pulmonary:* Pleurisy, dyspnea, cough, hemoptysis, chest pain (lower lobe pneumonia can cause thoracoabdominal pain)

  Examination.
  1. *General:* Have the patient fully recumbent, with abdomen exposed from rib cage to symphysis pubis. Flex the patient's knees slightly with a rolled sheet.

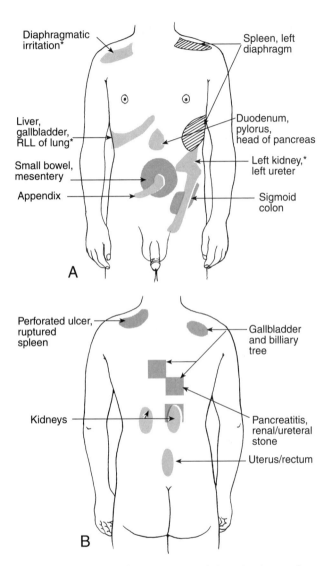

Figure 9.4 Common surface projections of visceral pain, not always true to locale. **A.** Anterior. *Asterisk* indicates symmetric finding is seen with involvement of opposite paired organ. **B.** Posterior.

2. *Inspection:* Watch the patient's *face* for discomfort, either spontaneous or from palpation.

     Seek generalized abdominal distension or localized bulging and focal discoloration. Discovery of peristaltic movement is facilitated by shining a light at a low transverse angle across the abdominal wall.

3. *Auscultation:* Check whether the firmly placed stethoscope produces less pain than palpating fingers. Seek absent or high-pitched bowel sounds, bruits, or rubs. Are there loud intermittent rushes associated with visible peristalsis or cramps?

4. *Percussion:* Seek excessive tympany, enlarged organs, excessive suprapubic dullness. Does percussion elicit pain or guarding?

5. *Palpation:* If there is localized pain, begin palpation in nonpainful quadrants and away from any visible bulges or discoloration. Start lightly. Seek tenderness, guarding, organ enlargement, mass, or fecal impaction producing abnormal firmness.

Does the patient guard; i.e., does the area immediately become tense and resistant? Is there *rigidity*? If so, is it localized or generalized? Can it be overcome by asking the patient to breathe slowly and deeply? Resistance that cannot be reduced by such simple relaxation maneuvers is involuntary. If generalized **involuntary guarding** prevents deep palpation, recognize that other assessment methods are needed. With regional voluntary guarding, the protected area can sometimes be assessed by palpating deeply from adjacent areas.

Rebound tenderness is elicited by sudden removal of palpation pressure. If pain is worst as and after pressure is released, **rebound tenderness** is present. Rebound can be direct (at the palpated site) or referred (remote from the area being palpated).

Small bowel obstruction in an incarcerated or strangulated **hernia** can be missed as the cause of acute abdominal pain; all potential hernial sites (Fig. 9.5) are systematically inspected and palpated.

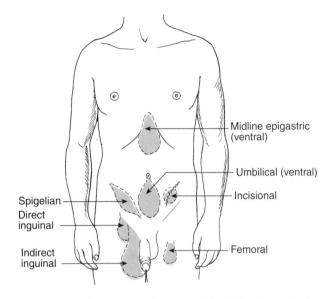

Figure 9.5 Sites of presentation of common abdominal and groin **hernias**.

If there is tenderness to palpation of the liver, have the patient inspire deeply while you press deeply below the liver edge (or the rib cage, if the liver is impalpable). Abrupt *arrest of respiration* when examining fingers contact the gallbladder region is a positive *Murphy's sign*.

Have the patient flex the thigh on the painful side, then attempt to extend it against the resistance of your hand. Pain deep in the pelvis produced by this *iliopsoas maneuver* (Fig. 9.6*A*) is a positive test. To assess for irritation over the obturator muscle area, have the patient flex the thigh on the affected side to 90°. Then fix the ankle and, with your other hand, externally rotate the hip by pulling the patient's knee laterally against resistance (Fig. 9.6*B*). Pelvic pain produced thereby is a positive *obturator test*.

6. *Other, indispensable:* Rectal examination is essential in evaluating abdominal pain, to seek tender sites, masses, and pelvic tenderness. In women, a full *bimanual pelvic* examination is mandatory as well,

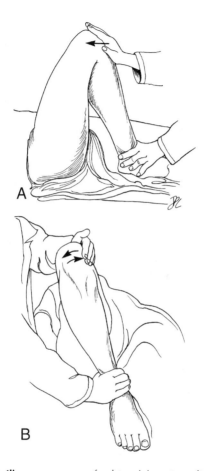

Figure 9.6 **A. Iliopsoas maneuver** for determining retroperitoneal irritation. Fix the patient's foot and ankle with your left hand as the patient attempts to extend his thigh against patellar pressure. **B.** Obturator maneuver. External and internal rotation of the flexed hip with the ankle fixed causes pain of irritated ipsilateral obturator muscle.

to determine whether internal genitalia or adjacent structures are the source of the pain. *Genital examination* is vital in assessing abdominal pain in men.

Interpretation. Causes of abdominal pain abound (Table 9.2). At the most serious end, involuntary resistance indicates peritoneal irritation. Rebound tenderness, whether direct or referred, also indicates peritoneal irritation.

Generalized distension of the acute abdomen suggests *ileus*, which may be metabolic as well as mechanical. Obstructed intestine eventually dilates as normal peristalsis ceases and smooth muscle paralysis sets in. Inflammation as in peritonitis, local ischemia, and lack of chemical substrates and mediators (e.g., in hypokalemia) can all produce ileus. When gas dilates the nonfunctioning segment, it becomes tympanitic. The distended, silent, tympanitic abdomen signals advanced ileus. A normal intestine may be silent in the patient on a respirator as a result of lack of air swallowing, but it does not become tympanitic.

With ileus, *rigidity* signifies **peritonitis**. Ileus without peritoneal signs such as rigidity or involuntary guarding suggests mechanical obstruction (but without perforation of a viscus) or some chemical derangement, including narcotic- and bed rest-induced **pseudo-obstruction** (Ogilvie's syndrome). Ileus plus loops of visibly dilated small intestine (ladder sign) suggests volvulus or ileocecal obstruction. Visibly distended large bowel points to distal colonic obstruction. A mass obstructing the finger on rectal examination announces a dramatic cause.

Jaundice, spider angiomata, and engorged abdominal wall veins in a patient with a distended, painful, tender abdomen raises the question of *spontaneous bacterial peritonitis.*

Visible peristalsis in the nondistended acute abdomen suggests *early intestinal obstruction* in the stage preceding ileus. Nausea and vomiting, the usual concomitants of small bowel obstruction, may not yet have supervened. Auscultation will reveal (*a*) loud rushes of bowel sounds separated by periods of silence or (*b*) generalized hyperactive bowel sounds.

Table 9.2
Acutely Painful Abdomen[a]

Symptoms and Signs	Considerations	Other Evidence
Central pain only	**Early appendicitis**	
	Small bowel obstruction	
	Acute pancreatitis	
	[Acute myocardial infarction]	
	[Pericarditis and pleuritis]	
	[Herpes zoster]	
	[Spontaneous bacterial peritonitis]	
Central pain with vascular collapse	Acute pancreatitis	Back and flank pain; vomiting; rigidity
	Acute mesenteric ischemia	Maroon stool
	Ruptured aortic aneurysm	Shock; radiation to groin/perineum; pulsatile mass
	Dissecting aortic hematoma	Often begins in chest and back; absent femoral pulses
	[Myocardial infarction]	Chest features
	Intra-abdominal hemorrhage	Abdominal distension; shortness of breath with shallow respirations
Pain, vomiting, and distension	**Small bowel obstruction**	Visible peristalsis common
	Early peritonitis	Increasing rigidity
Severe pain, shock, and general rigidity	Perforated viscus	Board-like rigidity, vomiting, distension
	Dissecting aortic hematoma	
	Ruptured aortic aneurysm	
LUQ pain and rigidity	Pancreatitis	Vomiting
	Perforated gastric ulcer	
	Splenic rupture	
	Acute upper urinary tract stone or infection	Sometimes dysuria and back pain
	[LLL pneumonia]	Chest features
RUQ pain and rigidity	[RLL pneumonia]	Chest features
	[Pleurisy]	Chest features
	Acute cholecystitis	Rigidity variable, Murphy's sign
	Leaking duodenal ulcer	
	Perforated/penetrating ulcer	

Table 9.2 *(continued)*
Acutely Painful Abdomen[a]

Symptoms and Signs	Considerations	Other Evidence
	Pancreatitis	Vomiting, rarely Cullen's sign
	Subphrenic appendix with appendicitis	
	Subphrenic abscess	
LLQ pain, tenderness, guarding	**Diverticulitis**	
	Pelvic peritonitis secondary to salpingitis	
	Ruptured ectopic pregnancy	
RLQ pain and rigidity	**Appendicitis with or without rupture**	
	Pelvic peritonitis secondary to salpingitis	
	Ruptured ectopic pregnancy	

[a]**Boldface**, common; [. . .], extra-abdominal etiologies; LLL, left lower lobe; RLL, right lower lobe.

In the painful, guarded abdomen, periumbilical blue-purple to greenish-yellow discoloration (Cullen's sign) or flank ecchymoses (Grey Turner's sign) indicate seepage of blood along tissue planes from *intraperitoneal* or *retroperitoneal hemorrhage*, classically in hemorrhagic pancreatitis but also in vascular catastrophes and other settings.

Intense pain in one flank, especially with radiation to the groin and vulva or penis and scrotum, is characteristic of **ureteral calculus**, in which examination of the abdomen is surprisingly normal, so much so that you may misinfer psychogenic pain.

Murphy's sign strongly suggests **acute cholecystitis**, unless a positive punch test of the liver (see below) has been misinterpreted.

A positive iliopsoas maneuver or obturator test indicates *irritation of the retroperitoneum* near the ipsilateral iliopsoas muscle.

EVALUATION OF DISTENSION

Goal. Determine the nature and cause of the process distending the abdomen or a portion of it.

Technique. Repeat all four modalities, seeking masses and ascites with especial vigilance.

If a bulge suggesting a hernia is present, use fingertips to define the rim of the defect through which it protrudes. By pressing gently against it, determine whether or not it is tender and can be reduced easily back into the abdominal cavity. *Do not force reduction of a painful, tender, or resistant herniation.* A bulge or break in the smooth contour that arises in the extraperitoneal wall can usually be partially surrounded by the examining fingers and will be definable as subcutaneous by becoming sharper when the patient lifts his head from the table, a maneuver that tenses the muscles beneath the mass.

Interpretation. Generalized distension without pain may reflect obesity, poor muscle tone, or the causes listed in Table 9.1.

Localized distension of the upper abdomen can be caused by gastric dilation resulting from outlet obstruction, gastroparesis, or prior surgery. An enlarged liver or a tumor of the upper abdominal organs can change the surface contour.

A uterus enlarged by pregnancy or neoplasm may distort the lower abdominal contour, as may a huge ovarian mass or a greatly distended urinary bladder. Cecal distension rarely creates the same finding. In the thin patient, a large accumulation of feces in the sigmoid colon is sometimes visible in the LLQ and may represent impaction or megacolon.

Discrete bulges on the surface of the abdomen can represent subcutaneous masses, hernias, or intra-abdominal masses. A mass that becomes *more prominent with muscle tensing* (raising the head) must be a *superficial structure* or a *herniation.* Such hernias are most common in the midline above the umbilicus, around the umbilicus, at the site of a surgical scar, or at the margins of the abdominal muscles (Fig. 9.5).

Generalized distension in the absence of ileus suggests ascites, discussed immediately below.

ASCITES EVALUATION

Goal. Determine whether the peritoneal cavity contains excess fluid, and if it does, characterize its cause and nature.

Technique. Signs suggestive of free fluid include bulging flanks and those cited below:

- *Shifting dullness:* This is a dynamic alteration of the percussion note as the patient's position changes. With the patient supine, the air-containing (resonant) bowel floats to the top of ascites, and so the flank is dull; when the patient rolls onto one side, the bowel assumes a new position, and the flank becomes resonant.

- *Fluid wave:* With the patient supine, hold one hand (the "receiving" hand) on one flank and press in with it. Tap the other hand sharply against the opposite flank while an assistant compresses the midabdomen. The "receiving" hand feels a wave of fluid driven by the other hand.

A large ovarian cyst may produce several false signs of ascites. The thin-walled, fluid-filled sac can distend the abdomen, evert the umbilicus, cause bulging of the flanks, and produce shifting dullness and a fluid wave. The percussion note, however, will be dull anteriorly. Some cysts transmit aortic pulsations; ascitic fluid dampens them.

Interpretation. The sensitivity of physical examination alone for detecting ascites is poor, but nihilism is not justified. Distinction from large ovarian cysts depends on the characteristics cited above.

LIVER EVALUATION

Technique. If you have difficulty defining the lower border of the patient's liver, try the *scratch test* (Fig. 9.7):

1. Auscultate just above the costal margin in the right midclavicular line.
2. Scratch one finger gently against the skin as you move it progressively cephalad along the right midclavicular line.
3. When the scratching finger crosses the liver edge, sound transmits more clearly through the solid organ.

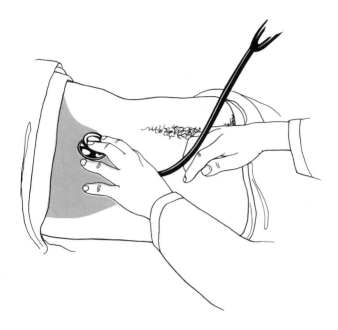

Figure 9.7 Scratch test for definition of an elusive liver margin.

4. Once the liver margin is identified, it is repalpated, and irregularities of contour or consistency are noted.

Seek tenderness to a *light* punch just above the right costal margin, 5 cm lateral to the midclavicular line.

Interpretation. An enlarged, smooth, nontender liver can harbor fatty infiltration, lymphoma or leukemia, infiltrative amyloid or hematopoiesis, primary or metastatic carcinoma, or parasitic infestation.

If an enlarged liver is tender, consider hepatitis, heart failure, hepatic venous obstruction, and bacterial or parasitic infection.

A *very hard liver* is specific, albeit insensitive, for neoplastic infiltration. Surface nodules are found in metastatic carcinoma and in some cirrhoses.

Tumors of the liver, both primary and metastatic, can produce diffuse enlargement or discrete masses contiguous with normal-feeling liver.

EVALUATION OF SPLENOMEGALY

Goal. Detect enlargement of the spleen and find its cause.

Technique. With the patient in the right lateral decubitus position, feel for the tip of the spleen:
1. Use your left hand to press the flank anteriorly from behind while you press your right hand beneath the cartilage of ribs 9–11.
2. The amount of spleen felt below the rib margin is measured in fingerbreadths to semiquantify organ size.
3. *Gently* assess a palpable spleen for tenderness and consistency. It is normally somewhat soft but, when enlarged, can become quite firm.
4. Further assess the area by moving to the patient's left side; keep the patient in the *right* lateral decubitus position.
5. Place both hands on the left costal border and "hook" your fingertips around the costal margin at the tip of ribs 9–11.
6. On deep inspiration, an enlarged spleen may tap your flexed fingers.
7. Percuss over the lowest intercostal space in the midaxillary line while the patient inhales and exhales slowly and deeply.

Interpretation. The spleen may harbor a host of infectious, hematologic, and infiltrative diseases. With upper abdominal or flank trauma and a tender, palpable spleen, consider subcapsular hematoma also.

Resonance during expiration, which is replaced by dullness in deep inspiration, strongly suggests splenomegaly.

EVALUATION OF ABDOMINAL MASSES

Goal. Detect masses, discriminate them from organomegaly, and determine their source and nature.

Technique.

1. Have the patient tense the abdominal wall muscles; contracted muscles cloak an intraperitoneal or retroperitoneal structure, which "disappears" with this maneuver. Unchanged or enhanced palpability with abdominal contraction localizes the mass to the abdominal wall.
2. Deep palpation is used to determine size, mobility, attachments, and movement with deep respiration.
3. Try to determine whether a mass is solid or cystic by percussion.
4. Palpate a mass to determine indentability.
5. A mass in the lower abdomen requires pelvic and rectal examinations to define the extent and organ of origin further once a distended urinary bladder has been ruled out.
6. *Auscultatory percussion* may help delineate bladder distension:
    a. Using your nondominant hand, hold the bell of the stethoscope in the midline immediately above the symphysis pubis.
    b. With a finger of your dominant hand, percuss the symphysis in a midline vertical plane beginning just below the umbilicus.
    c. When your percussing finger reaches the upper border of a urine-filled bladder, you will notice an abrupt increase in intensity of the transmitted sound heard through the bell.
7. When an enlarged kidney is suspected, attempt to "capture" it:
    a. Standing on the side to be examined, place your left hand posteriorly in the flank, parallel to the plane of the table.
    b. Palpate deeply anteriorly under the rib margins with your right hand, in a parallel plane.
    c. Have the patient inhale deeply, and press your hands toward each other. As the patient exhales, reduce inward pressure and feel the kidney slip between your hands.

      d. If there is a palpable kidney, palpate for irregularity of contour and for tenderness.

    Interpretation. A wide differential diagnosis obtains (Table 9.3).

Table 9.3
Commonest Abdominal Masses

Superficial and subcutaneous masses
  Fibromas, lipomas, and other innocuous masses
  Hernias

Intra-abdominal masses
  RUQ
    Hepatomegaly
    Inflammation of biliary tree
    Obstruction of biliary tree
    Tumors of right kidney
  LUQ
    Splenomegaly
    Tumors of left kidney
    Feces in splenic flexure of colon
    Gastric masses
    Pancreatic masses (rare)
  Epigastric
    Pancreatic cyst or tumor
    Neoplasm or infection of stomach, omentum, transverse colon,
      left lobe of liver
    Gastric outlet obstruction
    Aortic aneurysm
  RLQ
    Inflammation, abscess, or neoplasm of cecum or appendix
    Inflammation or tumor of right salpinx or ovary
  LLQ
    Inflammation or tumor of sigmoid colon, including diverticular
      abscess
    Fecal impaction of sigmoid colon
    Inflammation or tumor of left salpinx or ovary
  Midline lower abdomen
    Aortoiliac enlargement
    Bladder distension
    Enlargement of uterus from pregnancy or tumor

RUQ masses.
1. Think of the liver.
2. A mass on the inferior surface of the liver suggests gallbladder hydrops or carcinoma (acute cholecystitis is too tender for the patient to tolerate palpation).
3. A palpable nontender gallbladder suggests regional malignancy.
4. A polycystic right kidney, hydronephrosis, large renal cyst, or renal tumor can also produce a RUQ mass, as can a cancer of the hepatic flexure of the colon.

LUQ masses.
1. Splenomegaly
2. Tumors of the splenic flexure of the colon
3. Palpable left kidney: enlarged
4. Retroperitoneal mass

Epigastric mass.
1. Matted omentum
2. Pancreatic cancer or pseudocyst
3. Neoplasm of the stomach, liver, or transverse colon

RLQ mass.
1. Feces in cecum
2. Cecal carcinoma
3. Firm, mildly tender:
    a. Crohn's disease
    b. Periappendiceal abscess
    c. Granulomatous disease
4. Tubo-ovarian abscesses and neoplasms

LLQ mass.
1. Tubo-ovarian abscesses and neoplasms
2. Sigmoid colon:
    a. Diverticulitis with abscess formation
    b. Cancer
    c. Distension with feces, suggested by diagonal "sausage" shape and indentability by palpating finger

Suprapubic masses.
1. Distended urinary bladder
2. Uterine enlargement

EVALUATION OF ABDOMINAL VASCULAR ABNORMALITIES

Goal. Determine the origin and significance of abdominal vascular abnormalities.

Technique. When an **abdominal murmur** is heard, inch the stethoscope to determine the point of greatest intensity or whether the sound is transmitted cardiac sound. Assess systolic and diastolic components and direction(s) of radiation.

Interpretation. If the pulsation appears to be lateral, consider an aneurysm.

A murmur of **renal artery stenosis** may be audible in the midline but often radiates to or is best heard in a flank or even posteriorly; lateralization is unreliable, as is discrimination by physical examination between atherosclerotic and fibromuscular stenoses.

The test characteristics for **aortic aneurysm** discovery are discouraging: Aortic pulsations are impalpable in many persons. Overdiagnosis of aortic aneurysm is common when there are striking but normal pulsations. Many large aortic aneurysms are impalpable, particularly in the obese.

Most **innocent abdominal bruits** are confined to systole and are heard in the midline between the xiphoid and the umbilicus. They have low intensity and pitch. A bruit occasionally found in pancreatic carcinoma is usually sharply localized in the LUQ. Bruits from hepatic tumors are often loud and harsh and located directly over the liver; the combination of a hepatic rub and bruit is more specific than either alone for primary or metastatic liver cancer.

Absence or diminution of pulse in either or both femoral arteries points to obstructive disease in the aortoiliofemoral arterial system.

10

Limbs

Assessment of limbs follows anatomy, special principles (Table 10.1), and four functional systems.

Table 10.1
Principles of Limb Examination

Begin after completion of abdominal examination.
Have patient lie supine for initial inspection and palpation of anterior lower limbs and for partial assessment of hip joint.
Have patient sit for further lower limb examination and all of upper limb examination. A half-sheet covers the genitals.
As examination of each limb proceeds, work from proximal to distal.
Joint range of motion and neuromuscular assessments are combined by region.
If patient cannot **actively** perform a movement, attempt motion **passively,** i.e., move the joint in question for him. If neither you nor patient can put the joint through normal range of motion, stiffness suggests joint or periarticular disease.

- Upper limb
     Arterial, venous, and capillary circulation
     Lymphatic drainage
     Joints, tendons, muscles, and bones
          Shoulder
          Elbow
          Wrist
          Hand and fingers
     Peripheral nerves and muscles
- Lower limb
     Arterial, venous, and capillary circulation
     Lymphatic drainage
     Joints, tendons, muscles, and bones

Hip
Knee
Ankle and foot
Feet and toes
    Peripheral nerves and muscles
With each joint, tendon, muscle, and bone evaluation, range of motion assessment is described first, immediately followed by tests of pertinent musculature.

UPPER LIMB

Arterial, Venous, and Capillary Circulation

Goal. Evaluate the integrity of the regional and systemic vasculature and of tissue oxygen delivery.

Technique. **Pinch purpura** is sought by moderately firmly pinching the patient's arm.

Interpretation. If an ecchymosis develops at the site, there is arteriolar fragility. If only a few petechiae result, consider *cardiologist's purpura* (low-dose aspirin effect).

Technique. *Osler nodes* and *Janeway lesions*, seldom found, are sought by inspecting the hands, wrists, ankles, and feet. If unexplained macules, papules, or pustules are discovered, check for tenderness with a *gloved* finger.

Interpretation. Classically, Osler nodes are tender papules, and Janeway lesions are nontender macules. Both are red-purple.

Technique. To find an *elusive **brachial artery pulse***, push biceps tendon laterally (not deeper) to uncover the pulsation. If *reduced blood flow to one arm* is being pursued, *measure bilateral upper limb blood pressures;* inequalities on sphygmomanometry may be present even without pulse asymmetry. To seek a functional rather than a fixed cause for this *subclavian steal syndrome*, have the patient exercise both arms, and observe for symptoms of vertebrobasilar insufficiency.

Interpretation. Twenty-torr disparity between systolic blood pressure in one arm and that in the other suggests subclavian artery stenosis (see Table 10.2). Vertebrobasilar

Table 10.2
Causes of Diminished Radial Pulse and of Unilateral Decreased
Blood Pressure

Arterial stenosis proximal to the site that is being palpated
Prior arterial thrombosis, classically from radial artery
  catheterization
Acutely, **dissecting hematoma**
With 20-torr gradient in systolic blood pressure between one arm
  and other, **subclavian artery stenosis**

---

symptoms (dizziness, vertigo, extraocular palsies) on arm
exercise demonstrate subclavian steal syndrome.

    Technique. Test for *brachioradial delay* by feeling one
brachial pulse with one hand and the ipsilateral radial pulse
with your other hand. Attend to whether there is a perceptible time lag between the two.

    Interpretation. Brachioradial delay correlates with the
transaortic valvular systolic pressure gradient. Thus brachioradial delay can further characterize systolic ejection murmurs maximal at the right upper sternal border.

    Technique. The *ulnar pulse* is palpable on the lateral
(radial) aspect of the ulna, just proximal to the wrist. If you
are in doubt about whether you are feeling your own digital
pulsations or the patient's ulnar pulse, palpate your own
radial or carotid pulse simultaneously.

    Interpretation. If your own pulse is synchronous with
the "ulnar," both are yours; if it is not, you have the patient's
ulnar in hand. An absent ulnar pulse calls for **Allen's test** to
determine functional significance.

    Goal. Perform *Allen's test* to demonstrate adequacy of the
collateral flow to the hand via both the radial and ulnar systems, lest arterial instrumentation result in finger necrosis.

    Technique. Have the patient make a tight fist to squeeze
blood out of the palm. Now press very firmly on both the
radial and ulnar pulses, using both thumbs (Fig. 10.1), and
wait a few seconds. If the whitened palm "pinks up," pressure has been insufficient, and the test must be restarted.
Otherwise, release the ulnar artery and measure the time
needed for recoloring of the palm. Repeat the maneuver,
releasing only the radial artery this time.

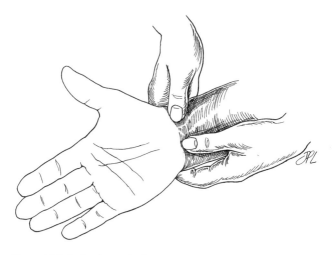

Figure 10.1 Early phase of Allen's test. Sustain firm pressure on both radial and ulnar arteries.

Interpretation. If color returns in less than 5 seconds, the palmar arch is intact. If it has not returned in 15 seconds, arteries of that hand should not be punctured or cannulated.

Technique. When *peripheral **cyanosis*** is observed, determine whether there is also central (oral or perioral) cyanosis, which constitutes an emergency. If it is not central, establish whether cyanosis is confined to the acral appendages (fingertips, toes, nipples, tip of penis) or extends proximally. When vasoconstriction is suspected as the cause of cyanosis localized to cold feet, rewarm the feet and then reinspect.

Interpretation. Central cyanosis suggests severe decarboxyhemoglobinemia of 5 g/dL or more of unsaturated hemoglobin in capillary (*not arterial*) blood, usually from marked cardiorespiratory dysfunction. There is a range of thresholds. For example, cyanosis becomes recognizable in some dark-pigmented persons at 6 g/dL.

Simple warming clears up normal vasoconstrictive cyanosis in cold feet but can accentuate central cyanosis.

Acrocyanosis can complicate pathologic vascular reactivity in Raynaud's disease, systemic lupus erythematosus, and systemic sclerosis. Acrocyanosis also occurs in low-flow states with high peripheral vascular resistance.

Lymphatic Drainage

Goals. Demonstrate the integrity and speed of regional drainage of lymph and the processing of same.

Technique. For the *epitrochlear nodes*, feel between the tendons of the biceps and triceps, with the patient's forearm supinated. For the *subhumeral nodes*, press firmly but not painfully high in the axilla against the humerus, and sweep back to front.

Interpretation. *Enlarged epitrochlear lymph nodes* suggest infection of the hand or forearm or a systemic nodal disorder. *Subhumeral nodes* may feel like "BBs" or "jelly beans" and may glide or pop under the fingertips. Their differential includes causes of epitrochlear lymphadenopathy and also breast disease.

Joints, Tendons, Muscles, and Bones

Goal. Demonstrate normality or disease of the regional locomotor apparatus.

SHOULDER

Technique. See Figure 10.2, *A–F*, for shoulder technique.
- *Abduction:* Have the patient raise his arms laterally until his fingers touch above his head. Ask him to lower both arms slowly. Observe whether his arm drops spontaneously after he has lowered it to 45°, with or without a nudge to increase the stress.
- *Adduction:* Have the patient move each arm across the front of his body as far as possible.
- *Flexion:* Have the patient "reach for the basket"—as far anterosuperiorly as possible.
- *Internal rotation:* Have the patient clasp his hands together behind his lower back.
- *External rotation:* Have the patient clasp his hands together behind his head.

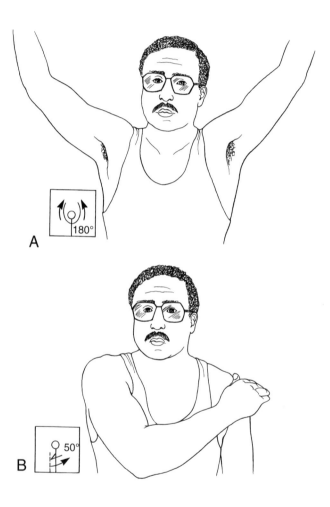

Figure 10.2 Range of motion of shoulder. **A.** Abduction: arms raised from sides. **B.** Adduction.

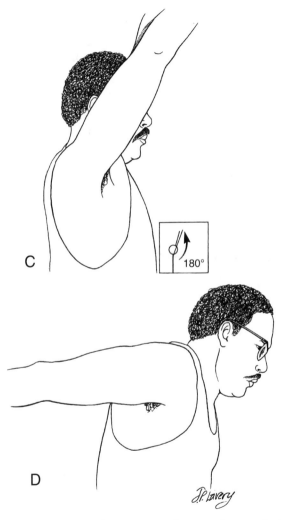

Figure 10.2—continued **C.** Flexion. Endpoint similar to endpoint of abduction. **D.** Extension.

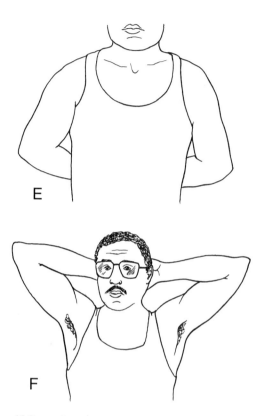

Figure 10.2—continued **E.** Internal rotation: hands clasped behind back. **F.** External rotation: hands clasped behind head.

- Look hard at the shoulders, individually and then together, from front and then back, fully exposed.
- Functional tests include the Apley scratch test (Table 10.3).
  Interpretation.
- *Reduction in active range of motion:* Repeat as passive range of motion.
- *Reduction of power:* Suggests disorders of local structures, including joints with pain, or of central connections

Table 10.3
Apley Scratch Test

Patient reaches hand behind head and touches ("scratches")
  superomedial angle of opposite scapula (lost with *defective abduction
  and external rotation*).
Patient reaches in front of chest to rest hand on opposite shoulder (lost
  with *decreased internal rotation and adduction*).
Patient reaches behind back to touch inferior angle of opposite scapula
  (lost with *decreased internal rotation and adduction*).

(see Table 10.4, as for movement of other upper
limb joints).

- *Normal abduction strength testing*, i.e., a normal drop-
  arm test: Excludes significant **rotator cuff tears.**
- *Unilateral dropped shoulder*
    Dislocation: Humeral tuberosity is displaced for-
    ward, and an indentation is seen just beneath.

Table 10.4
Muscle and Nerve Control of Upper Limb Joint Motion

	Motion	Muscles	Innervation	
			Nerve	Cord Segment
Shoulder	Elevation	Levator scapulae		C3–C5
		Trapezius	Cranial nerve XI	
	Abduction	Deltoid	Axillary	C5–C6
		Supraspinatus	Suprascapular	C4–C6
	Adduction	Pectoralis major	Medial and lateral pectoral	C5–T1
	Flexion	Coracobrachialis	Musculocutaneous	C6–C7
		Anterior deltoid	Axillary	C5–C6
	Extension	Latissimus dorsi	Subscapular	C5–C8
		Teres major		
	External rotation	Infraspinatus	Suprascapular	C5–C6
	Internal rotation	Subscapularis	Subscapular	C5–C8
		Teres major		
		Latissimus dorsi		
Elbow	Flexion	Biceps, brachialis	Musculocutaneous	C5–C6
	Extension	Triceps	Radial	C6–T1
	Supination of forearm	Biceps, supinator	Radial	C5–C7
	Pronation of forearm	Pronator teres	Median	C6–C7

Table 10.4 (continued)
Muscle and Nerve Control of Upper Limb Joint Motion

	Motion	Muscles	Innervation	
			Nerve	Cord Segment
Wrist	Flexion	Flexor carpi radiali	Median	C6–C8
		Flexor carpi ulnaris	Ulnar	C7–T1
	Extension	Extensor carpi radialis longus	Radial	C5–C8
		Extensor carpi ulnaris	Radial	C6–C8
Finger	Flexion	PIP joints: flexor digitorum super-ficialis, profundus[a]	Median	C7–T1
		MCP joints: flexor digitorum brevis, lumbricals[a]	Median Ulnar	C6–T1 C8–T1
		Distal phalanges: flexor digitorum profundus	Median Ulnar	C7–T1 C8–T1
	Extension	Extensor digitorum extensors to indi-vidual fingers	Radial	C6—C8
	Abduction	First dorsal interosseous, abductor digiti	Ulnar	C8–T1
	Adduction	Palmar interossei	Ulnar	C8–T1
Thumb	Abduction	Abductor pollicis brevis	Median	C6–T1
	Adduction	Adductor pollicis	Ulnar	C8–T1
	Flexion	Flexor pollicis brevis	Median	C8–T1
	Extension	Extensor pollicis longus and brevis	Radial	C6–C8
	Opposition of thumb and fifth finger	Opponens pollicis Opponens digiti minimi	Median Ulnar	C6–T1 C8–T1

[a]PIP, proximal interphalangeal; and MCP, metacarpophalangeal.

Reduced abductor tone.
- *Loss of convexity of shoulder:* Suggests atrophy of the deltoid muscle, often with prominence of the humerus.
- *Unilateral prominent clavicle:* Suggests **Paget's disease of bone,** sometimes misinterpreted as dislocation, bone neoplasm, or supraclavicular lymphadenopathy.

ELBOW

Technique.

- *Flexion:* Have the patient bend his elbow maximally; then say to him, "Don't let me straighten your arm."
- *Extension:* Have the patient fully straighten his elbow, with his arm at his side; then say to him, "Don't let me bend your arm." Complete extension is avoided to preclude locking.
- *Supination:* With forearms resting in his lap, have the patient turn the palms of his hands toward the ceiling.
- *Pronation:* With forearms resting in his lap, have the patient turn the palms of his hands toward his lap.
- *Angle of elbow:* Look at the carrying angle of the elbow, normally about 10° lateral (valgus) to the long axis of the upper arm with the limb in anatomic position.
- *Palpation for effusion:* Feel for somewhat indistinct soft-tissue fullness between the lateral epicondyle, proximal end of the radius, and the olecranon. If it is found, distinguish it from a more superficial fluid-filled bursal swelling directly over the olecranon and from subcutaneous solid masses.
- *Coen's test:* Hold the patient's proximal forearm, then have him make a fist and extend his wrist against your flexing pressure. Inquire about sudden severe pain. If the patient feels pain, ask where, being careful not to suggest an answer.

Interpretation.

- *Reduction in active range of motion:* Repeat as passive range of motion.
- *Reduction of power:* Suggests disorders of local structures, including joints with pain, or of central connections.
- *Increased carrying angle:* Suggests an old epicondylar fracture or, frequently, **rheumatoid arthritis.**
- *Effusion in elbow joint.*
    Any *inflammatory arthritis.*
    Superficial, localized *olecranon bursitis* fluid accumulations are common in gout.
    Subcutaneous rheumatoid nodules: Feel firmer than these fluid collections, with less "give."

- *Positive Coen's test*, with pain felt not at wrist but at elbow: Suggests lateral epicondylitis or radiohumeral bursitis (tennis elbow).

Technique. Feel for nontender subcutaneous nodules near bony prominences, especially over the elbow and the back of the forearm.

Interpretation.

Subcutaneous nodules
  Rheumatoid arthritis
  Gout
  Systemic lupus erythematosus
  Acute rheumatic fever
  Sarcoidosis
  Mimics
    Xanthomas, sometimes larger than rheumatoid nodules
    Epidermal inclusion cysts (sebaceous cysts), which indent, often show an overlying pore, and feel somewhat "squishy"
    Ganglion cysts, which are usually tender and located on the dorsum of the wrist or fingers, with no pore

WRIST

Technique.
- *Extension of wrist:* Have the patient elevate the back of his hand toward his wrist; with the wrist thus hyperextended, have the patient resist attempts to return it to a neutral position.
- *Flexion of wrist:* Have the patient bend his palm toward his wrist; then have the patient resist attempts to return it to a neutral position.

Interpretation.
- *Reduction in active range of motion:* Repeat as passive range of motion.
- *Reduction of power:* Suggests disorders of local structures, including joints with pain, or of central connections.

HAND AND FINGERS

Technique.

1. For screening (see also Table 10.5), perform the following:

Table 10.5
Advanced Hand Screen (Done on Each Hand Separately)

Make a tight fist.
Pick up a small object from a flat surface.
Squeeze two of examiner's fingers firmly.

---

  a. Ask the patient to spread his fingers apart and bring them back together, with his wrists in a neutral position.
  b. Then have him make a fist such that you can observe flexion of each metacarpophalangeal joint and each group of interphalangeal joints.
  c. Have the patient grasp, squeeze, and hold the first two fingers of your hands in his grip.
  d. Have the patient pick up a small object.
2. Observe the patient's hands in the rest position, which normally shows slight flexion of all joints beyond the wrist.
3. To see ulnar deviation, have the patient lay both hands flat next to each other in his lap, with his palms down. Are his hands as a whole or any digits deviated "valgus fashion" to the ulnar side? Ascertain whether any of the metacarpophalangeal joints are selectively enlarged.
4. If the screening examination is positive, observe whether the patient's knuckles, whether at rest or making a fist, stand out from adjacent soft tissue. Confirm metacarpophalangeal joint inflammation by noting (*a*) tenderness on compression or warmth or (*b*) a wince on handshake.
5. Take one more look at the hands as a whole and one more feel of them.

Interpretation.

1. If the patient can shake hands firmly and make a normally formed tight fist and if hands lying flat on a table look normal, significant hand arthritis is unlikely.

2. If the test is completed without functional defect, pain, or visible deformity, further evaluation is seldom indicated.

3. A finger that remains extended when its mates are not must have damaged or disrupted flexor tendons. One that is *more* flexed than others likely has a flexion contracture; when there is an associated palmar nodule, it is known as *Dupuytren's contracture*.

4. Ulnar deviation is characteristic of rheumatoid arthritis, as are certain patterns of joint deformity (Table 10.6). With these, both active range of motion

Table 10.6
Finger Deformities

Deformity	Pattern
Swan-neck	Hyperextension of proximal interphalangeal and flexion of distal interphalangeal joint. Analogous process in thumb lacks "swan's head" because of one less phalanx.
Boutonnière	Opposite pattern, flexion of proximal inter-phalangeal, hyperextension of distal inter-phalangeal. Resembles knuckle protruding through collar buttonhole.
Metacarpophalangeal arthritis	Soft tissue diffusely swollen over dorsum of hand.
Dorsal knuckle pads	Thickening of dorsum of proximal interpha-langeal joints (not of metacarpophalangeal joints).

and passive range of motion of affected joints are diminished, as is hand strength.

5. Knuckle *pads* can be seen with any arthritis. *Erythematous* cutaneous thickening over the dorsum of the metacarpophalangeal joints is, how-ever, *Gottron's sign* of dermatomyositis. Knuckles that fail to stand out in a normal fashion constitute a

knuckle sign, indicating metacarpophalangeal arthritis unless there is swelling of the entire dorsum of the hand.

6. Rock-hard "joint" enlargement usually means abnormal exposure of bone as a result of movement of bone on bone (subluxation) or alterations in vectors of tendon-muscle tension. Soft swellings are usually fluid, i.e., joint effusion. Intermediate "boggy" consis-tency means fluid or overgrowth of synovial tissue.

7. Fusiform swellings of proximal interphalangeal joints (PIPs):
   a. *Rheumatoid arthritis.*
   b. When confined to the third and fourth fingers, consider *hemochromatosis arthropathy.*

8. Bony enlargement of PIPs **(Bouchard's nodes):**
   a. Rheumatoid arthritis.
   b. **Osteoarthrosis.**
   c. Posttraumatic change.
   d. Infection (rare).

9. Distal interphalangeal joint enlargement, **Heberden's nodes:**
   a. Osteoarthrosis.

   b. Psoriatic arthritis. Prominent pitting in fingernails supports psoriasis. Both processes can produce considerable subluxation of distal phalanx on middle phalanx.

Goal. Using *Finkelstein's test,* seek de Quervain's chronic stenosing tenosynovitis of two thumb abductors and extensors.

Technique. Have the patient fold a painful thumb into its palm and then curl its ipsilateral fingers around it. Stabilize this forearm with one hand and push it toward its ulnar side to stretch the tendon in question. Ask the patient about symptoms produced by the maneuver.

Interpretation. A *positive Finkelstein's* test consists of sharp pain in the radial aspect of the wrist and dorsal forearm at the radial side of the base of the thenar eminence.

Peripheral Nerves and Muscles

Goal. Evaluate the integrity of the regional and systemic neuromuscular apparatus.

LIMB TREMOR

Tremor is more often spotted in the hands than elsewhere. Follow up as indicated in Table 10.7.

Table 10.7
Tremor Evaluation

Most proximal point of spontaneous occurrence?
Symmetrical?
Abnormal involuntary movements elsewhere (other limbs, trunk, jaw, lips, tongue, cheeks, face).
Does purposeful movement abolish tremor?
Romberg sign? Nystagmus?
Do amplitude, frequency, duration, force change with emotion?
Have patient bring hands close to face.
Family history? Gait? Mental status?
Cogwheeling?
Facies?
Speech?

Goal. Evaluate further for *basal nuclear disease*, prototypically *parkinsonism*, and other disorders as the cause of an observed tremor.

Technique. To bring out *cogwheel rigidity*, have the patient draw a circle in the air with the hand whose wrist is not being passively flexed and extended.

Interpretation. Consider **parkinsonism** with tremor, and also think of drug-induced parkinsonism, cerebellar disease, and essential tremor. Asymmetry does not rule out parkinsonism, nor does absence of associated features. Abnormal oral movements are especially common in tardive dyskinesia. Rest tremor suggests noncerebellar disease, whereas intention tremor is characteristic of **cerebellar disease**. Nystagmus or a positive Romberg test supports a cerebellar origin. Emotional exacerbation of tremor does not implicate a psychosomatic component.

Other Upper Limb Tests

Goal. Detect weakness of the serratus anterior muscle.

Technique. Observe the patient's scapula at rest. Then perform the *push-off test*. Have the patient stand facing a wall at a distance of about 30 cm. Have him place both hands flat against wall, with his elbows outward, and attempt to push himself away from the wall. Watch for scapular winging, i.e., movement of the medial half of the scapula posteriorly.

Interpretation. The winged scapula demonstrates serratus anterior muscle weakness, often from C5–C7 damage, e.g., from poliomyelitis.

Goal. Assess *median nerve problems*, e.g., carpal tunnel syndrome, especially with compatible sensory abnormalities and thenar wasting or weakness.

Technique. Have the patient flex his wrists in an inverted prayer attitude maximally for one full minute to elicit *Phelan's sign*.

Interpretation. Phelan's sign is occurrence of electric pain or tingling elicited with this maneuver. The positive and negative predictive values of Phelan's sign remain to be established, whereas those of the related Tinel's sign are unsatisfactory.

Goal. Study *intrinsic hand muscles*.

Technique. Inspect the hollows and ridges of the hand.

Interpretation. Interosseous atrophy is recognized by visible reduction in tissue between bones.

Goal. Test *finger abduction*.

Technique. Have the patient extend his wrist and metacarpal joints and abduct his four fingers very slightly. Encircle his four fingers between your thumb and index finger, and have the patient try to break your hold.

Interpretation. Weak finger abduction implicates dorsal interosseous muscles, the abductor digiti minimi muscle, and the ulnar nerve, C8 or T1.

Goal. Seek asterixis as evidence of metabolic encephalopathy.

Technique. *Asterixis* is a variably rhythmic failure to maintain voluntary muscular contraction. Elicitation requires cooperation; *the patient who is markedly stuporous cannot complete the test.* Ask the patient to pronate his forearms, extend his elbows, spread his fingers slightly, and hyperextend both his wrists "as though you are a cop stopping traffic for a full minute."

Interpretation. Abnormal response is a "flap" of both hands, whereby hyperextension is involuntarily lost and quickly involuntarily regained.

This may appear rhythmic or more random and is slower than tremor. Asterixis correlates with metabolic encephalopathy, e.g., from cirrhosis with impending liver failure, uremia, or ventilatory failure with hypercarbia, severe electrolyte imbalances, iatrogenic overdoses, and several kinds of poisoning and even rarely in heart failure and septicemia.

Unilateral asterixis is rarely seen in disorders of the midbrain.

LOWER LIMB

Arterial, Venous, and Capillary Circulation

Goals. Evaluate the integrity of the regional and systemic vasculature and of tissue oxygen delivery.

Technique. Find the *popliteal pulse* by slightly passively flexing the knee, placing fingers deep in the popliteal space (Fig. 10.3). Only the pulsation is felt, not the arterial wall.

Feel the *dorsalis pedis* in the space between the tendons to the hallux and the second toe; if having trouble, move proximally or distally, since its maximal force may be anywhere from the base of the toes to the front of the ankle. When the *posterior tibial pulse* is difficult to feel, search throughout the space behind the medial malleolus and anterior to the tendo Achillis; try passive dorsiflexion of the ankle, using your opposite hand.

Interpretation. A significant minority of healthy persons have nonpalpable dorsalis pedis pulses, and a smaller number have no locatable posterior tibial pulsation. Normal foot temperature, skin color, and hair distribution suggest this situation. In aged patients, both foot pulses are frequently impalpable; if the patient is free of claudication, foot ulcers, and trophic change, no action is needed.

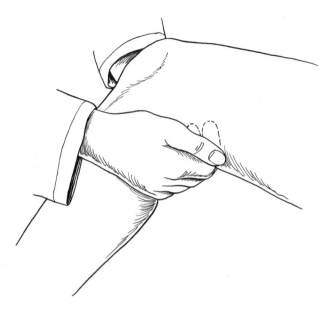

Figure 10.3 Palpable popliteal artery pulse, deep in popliteal fossa.

Goal. Using *Buerger's test*, search for subtle **arterial insufficiency of the leg.**

Technique. Passively raise the supine patient's leg just as for straight-leg raising. Observe for blanching on elevation, especially on the sole of the foot, and for reactive erythema over the dorsum of the foot on relowering the limb.

Interpretation. Blanching on elevation—a positive Buerger's test—indicates major arterial stenosis. It suggests severe ischemia and more distal limb artery disease. It is usually accompanied by reactive erythema on relowering. *Permanent* erythema over the feet in arterial insufficiency is *chronic erythromelia.*

Technique. In seeking to explain a leg with erythema that does not fit the above patterns, inquire about previous injury and about pain brought on by warmth or dependency and relieved by elevation or removal of coverings. Observe skin color with the leg in dependent, supine, and elevated positions.

Interpretation. **Reflex sympathetic dystrophy** produces pain, erythema, blanching, edema, and smooth shiny skin after an injury, sometimes after a long intervening delay. Settings include prior fracture, gunshot wound, or motor vehicle crash, which also predispose to venous injury, cellulitis, and osteomyelitis.

In erythromelalgia (erythermalgia), skin appears normal at baseline but turns deep red and painful with warming or dependency. Most patients with obstructive arterial disease experience relief with legs hanging, but this position is most uncomfortable in erythromelalgia. Skin warmth and absence of claudication support erythromelalgia, as does a negative Buerger's test.

Technique. For **edema** evaluation, see Table 10.8. For the approach to the **acutely painful, swollen leg,** see Table 10.9.

Table 10.8
Features to Look for in Edema Evaluation

Chronic venous insufficiency?
Lymphadenopathy at apex (groin, axilla)?
Symmetry?
Inflammatory features (erythema, marked tenderness, heat)? Red streaks at proximal margin?
Known stimulus, e.g., bee sting?
Smooth or bumpy?
Gravitational?
Effect of use of limb?
"Pitting" type, i.e., retains indentations made by a prodding fingertip applied for 10 seconds?
Most proximal point of pitting (separate from most proximal point of visible swelling)?
Measured circumference of the limb and its mate?
Skin shiny (usual with tense edema), atrophic, hyperkeratotic, scaly?

In seeking **chronic venous insufficiency** of the lower limb, have the patient stand upright for a full minute. For a weak patient, let him rest his buttocks against a table with hips minimally flexed. External rotation of the hip exposes ectatic veins on the medial aspect of the thigh and leg.

Table 10.9
Features in Assessing Acutely Painful, Swollen Leg

Finding	Suspect
No helpful findings	Need to exclude **deep venous thrombosis**
Red, hot, tender	**Cellulitis** likely
Crescent of extravasated blood near medial malleolus	Ruptured Baker's cyst, especially if known arthritis of knee
Onset during vigorous exercise	Ruptured plantaris longus tendon
Prior deep venous thrombosis in limb	Recurrent thrombosis or flare-up of **postphlebitic syndrome**
Therapeutically or supratherapeutically anticoagulated	Hemorrhage into calf—look for faint blue-purple to greenish discoloration
HIV seropositivity, especially with Kaposi's sarcoma	Hyperalgesic pseudothrombophlebitis

Interpretation. A differential diagnosis of edema appears in Table 10.10. Varicose veins produce soft bulges just under the skin that are variably mobile and usually nontender and compressible unless secondarily thrombosed. They are often bluish. Edema sometimes accompanies them. There may be an associated rusty spotting from hemosiderin. When skin is scaly, thickened, and erythematous as well as brown-flecked, it is *dermatitis venosa*; when it is also indurated, it is *dermatoliposclerosis*.

Lymphatic Drainage

Goal. Evaluate the integrity and speed of regional drainage of lymph.

Technique.
- *Popliteal nodes:* Passively flex the knee with the patient prone; probe deep in the popliteal fossa.
- *Inguinofemoral lymph nodes:* Feel for a diagonal group along the inguinal ligament inferomedially and vertically medial to the femoral vein.

Interpretation.
- Popliteal lymph nodes can enlarge with inflammation of the feet but are rarely felt.

Table 10.10
Causes of Edema

Venous hypertension
  Local causes
    Chronic venous insufficiency
    Acute venous insufficiency, with venous thrombosis
    Venous obstruction, including at pelvis, at pericardium, at venae
      cavae
  Congestive heart failure
Leaky capillaries
  Local inflammation, e.g., cellulitis
  Vasculitides
Hypoalbuminemia
  Cirrhosis, with synthetic failure
  Nutritional (cachexia and kwashiorkor)
  Nephrotic
  Protein-losing enteropathies
Lymphedema
  Local
  Inguinal, pelvic, axillary, or at cisterna chyli or thoracic duct
Adipose pseudoedema
Myxedema
Angioedema
Idiopathic edema

- Innocuous inguinal node enlargement is common; some times suppuration—characteristically on the foot—is responsible, or even malignancy, typically lymphoma and seldom in isolation.

Technique. Cellulitis evaluation: Inspect, palpate, and measure both limb circumference and the borders of erythema. *Lymphangitic streaking* is sought by scrutinizing the lymphatic course between the affected part and its nodal drainage at the groin or axilla, making the most of wide exposure and good lighting.

Interpretation. Ominous features in cellulitis are listed in Table 10.11. Lymphangitic streaking is specific but not sensitive for virulent bacterial cellulitides and lymphangitides. Lymphangitic streaking is *not* ordinarily seen when a melanoma, for instance, spreads to regional lymph nodes.

Table 10.11
Ominous Clinical Features in Cellulitis

Blackened skin or devitalization
Ulcer that develops or enlarges during course of treatment
Brown or foul discharge
Softening of affected area
Sloughing of skin
Palpable gas, i.e., crepitus
Suppuration of lymph nodes

Joints, Tendons, Muscles, and Bones

Goal. Evaluate the integrity of the regional locomotor apparatus.

INTEGRATED LOWER LIMB FUNCTION

Technique and interpretation. See Table 10.12, **Tinetti Functional Test**.

HIP

Technique. With the patient supine, perform the following:
- *Flexion:* With the patient's knee extended, have him elevate his leg as far as possible off the table and resist replacement of it onto the table.
- *Extension:* Done with lower back examination.
- *External rotation:* (For internal and external rotation testing, the knee must stay flexed to 45°.) Rotate the patient's hip externally (laterally); then have the patient maintain this position against your pulling it toward midline.
- *Internal rotation:* With the patient's knee flexed at 45°, rotate his hip somewhat internally (medially); then have the patient maintain this position against your attempt to externally rotate the hip.
- *Abduction:* With the patient supine and the limb straight, have the patient move the limb laterally; then have him resist your attempt to return it to midline.
- *Adduction:* With the limb straight, have the patient cross it medially over opposite lower limb; then have him resist your attempt to forcibly abduct it.

Table 10.12
Tinetti Functional Test

Performance: Patient arises, walks along a straight path (indicated by pointing), turns around, returns, and sits down again in a chair. Patient employs his regular shoes, hearing aid, eyeglasses, and cane or walker and traverses the longest available pathway free of obstacles. Observe patient's ability to arise from a chair, the step height, smoothness and ease of turning, and ability to sit down again smoothly and on target.

Abnormal arising from a chair
  Interpretation criteria: Hesitant or pushes off with arms, or shuffles buttocks forward to arise, or shows unsteadiness on first standing.
  Causes: Decreased knee extension, poor proprioceptive and cerebellar functions.

Problems with step height
  Interpretation criteria: Scraping, shuffling, or excess raising of foot (tip of toe lifted more than 5 cm above floor in midstride).
  Causes: Decreased hip or knee strength, reduced near vision, or proprioceptive deficit at PIPs of toes.

Turning deficits
  Interpretation criteria: Stopping completely before turning, staggering, swaying, and grabbing an object for support.
  Causes: Similar step-height deficits.

Abnormal sitting down in a chair
  Interpretation criteria: Plopping in chair or landing off center.
  Causes: Decreased hip flexion and decreased knee flexion.

Interpretation.
- *Reduction in active range of motion:* Repeat as passive range of motion.
- *Reduction of power:* Disorders of local structures, including joints with pain, or of central connections. See Table 10.13, as for other joint movements in the lower limb.

  Goal. Assess gluteus medius strength.

  Technique. The *Trendelenburg test* consists of observing from behind and looking at dimples over the posterior superior iliac spines (Fig. 10.4). With weight borne equally on both legs, both buttocks should be at the same level. Have the patient stand on one leg; observe for elevation of the opposite hemipelvis.

  Interpretation. A positive Trendelenburg test, i.e., sagging of the unsupported buttock or failure of elevation, sug-

Table 10.13
Muscle and Nerve Control of Lower Limb Joint Motion

	Motion	Muscles	Innervation	
			Nerve	Cord Segment
Hip	Flexion	Iliopsoas	Lumbar branches, femoral	T12–L4
	Extension	Gluteus maximus "Hamstrings"	Inferior gluteal, sciatic branches	L5–S2 L4–S3
	External rotation	Obturator *Quadratus* femoris	Obturator	L2–L4
	Internal rotation	Gluteus medius Gluteus minimus	Superior gluteal	L4–S1
	Abduction	Gluteus medius Gluteus minimus	Superior gluteal	L4–S1
	Adduction	Adductors Gracilis	Obturator	L2–L4
Knee	Flexion	"Hamstring"	Sciatic branches	L4–S3
	Extension	*Quadriceps* femoris	Femoral	L2–L4
Ankle	Dorsiflexion	Tibialis anterior	Deep peroneal	L4–S1
	Plantar flexion	Gastrocnemius Soleus	Femoral	L2–L4
	Supination of foot	Tibialis anterior Tibialis posterior	Deep peroneal Tibial	L4–S1 L5–S2
	Pronation of foot	Long extensor of digits	Deep and superficial peroneal	L4–S1
Toes	Flexion	Flexor hallucis longus and brevis Flexor digitorum longus	Tibial	L5–S2
	Extension	Extensor hallucis longus, extensor digitorum longus	Deep peroneal	L4–S1

gests weakness of the ipsilateral gluteus medius muscle. Frequently, gait will reflect this with a peculiar *lurch.* Associated weakness of hip abduction may or may not be evident on resistance testing.

Goal. Unmask occult *flexion contracture of hip.*

Technique. *Thomas' test:* Have the patient lie supine, with both legs adducted to midline. Inspect for excessive hollow between the superior aspect of the buttock and the small of the back. The hip contralateral to a suspected con-

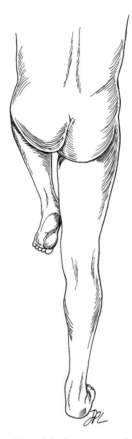

Figure 10.4 Normal Trendelenburg test result. Buttock does not sag with ipsilateral hip.

tracture is flexed fully up onto the trunk. This flattens the lumbar spine and stabilizes the pelvis, eliminating compensatory lordosis and bringing out hidden flexion contracture contralaterally.

Interpretation. An enlarged "hollow" at the small of the back increases the specificity of Thomas' test. An abnormal test consists of uncovering flexion of one hip when the other is maximally flexed.

Goal. Detect **gait** abnormalities, both for functional insight and apropos **back and hip pain**.

Technique. Observe gait closely, preferably without the patient being aware. Watch regular forward gait, turns, walking on heels, walking on toes, and walking in tandem. **Antalgic gait** suggests stepping on a tack, as one tries to abbreviate the weight-bearing phase. Another abnormal gait is *lurching gait,* whereby the pelvis falls when it is expected to rise.

Interpretation. Antalgic gait (favoring one leg) is seen in fracture, muscular overuse, thrombophlebitis, arthritides, foot disorders, etc. Lurching gait suggests weakness of the gluteus medius muscle.

KNEE

Goal. Assess the function, comfort, and prospect of fluid in the joint.

Technique.

- *Flexion:* (Partly checked during hip examination.) Have the patient resist your attempt to straighten the flexed knee.
- *Extension:* Have the patient straighten his leg. Then, with the knee barely flexed (170°), place one palm on the patient's thigh, and have the patient resist your attempt to flex the knee further.
- Assess the knee in the weight-bearing rest position.
- *Knee effusion detection:* See Table 10.14.

Interpretation.

- *Reduction in active range of motion:* Repeat as passive range of motion.
- *Reduction of power:* Disorders of local structures, including joints with pain, or of central connections.
- *Knock-knee* is genu valgum; the opposite deformity, *bowleg,* is genu varum. The effect of either deformity on musculoskeletal function is variable. *Genu recurvatum,* bent-back knee, creates inefficient gait.

Goal. Assess cruciate ligament integrity.

Table 10.14
Knee Effusion Detection

Have patient lie supine, with knee fully extended and quadriceps muscle relaxed.

Inspect for deformity, e.g., obliteration of normal indentations just medial and lateral to the patella.

Ballottement (tap test): Press suprapatellar pouch with one hand; push patella sharply posteriorly with your other hand; quickly release. With effusion, fluid wave rebounds from edges of joint cavity, and patella pops back up against examining fingers.

Bulge test: Squeeze suprapatellar pouch to milk fluid out of the medial part of the cavity. Push in just medial to the patella, creating a small concavity there. Then briskly stroke the lateral aspect, causing fullness to bulge outward on the medial side.

Fluctuation test: Squeeze suprapatellar pouch and rock fluid from medial to lateral side of patella and back again.

Mann's test: Observe, from side, hollows just lateral to patellar ligament with knee slightly flexed. With further flexion, hollow fills in. If excess fluid is present in knee, point of filling in is reached sooner.

Technique. *Knee draw(er) tests:*

1. Have the patient lie supine, with hips and knees flexed 90° and feet flat on the examination table.
2. Stabilize the foot on the side being tested by sitting on it sidesaddle.
3. Place both your hands around the knee in question, with your fingers in the popliteal fossa and your thumbs on the medial and lateral sides of the knee joint.
4. Draw the tibia forward, noting if it budges forward more than a few degrees from under the femur or more than on the opposite side.
5. Then push the tibia back, not only to the base position but also, if it will go, farther back under the femur.

Interpretation. Side-to-side comparison is requisite. Excess mobility of the tibia on the femur signifies cruciate ligament tear. Forward laxity is the *anterior draw sign* of a torn anterior cruciate ligament. Backward laxity behind rest position is the *posterior draw sign* from the rarer torn posterior cruciate ligament.

ANKLE AND FOOT

Technique.
- *Dorsiflexion:* Have the supine patient point both feet back at his head; then have him maintain dorsiflexion against your attempt to force his forefoot toward the floor.
- *Plantar flexion:* Tell the patient to "step on gas pedal"; then have him maintain plantar flexion against your attempt to dorsiflex his foot.
- *Inversion and eversion:* Stabilize the patient's leg above the ankle and have him rotate the sole of one foot away from his other foot (eversion) and then toward his other foot (inversion).
- *Plantar flexion of toes:* Have the patient curl his toes toward the sole; then have him resist your straightening them.
- *Extension of hallux:* While you stabilize the patient's foot in moderate plantar flexion, have him extend the great toe toward his chin; then have him resist your attempt to flex the extended great toe.

Interpretation.
- *Reduction in active range of motion:* Repeat as passive range of motion.
- *Reduction of power:* Disorders of local structures, including joints with pain, or of central connections.

Technique. To assess for **Charcot's joints**, see Table 10.15.

Interpretation. Charcot's joints result from neuropathic arthropathy, often at the ankle and often due to diabetic peripheral neuropathy.

Table 10.15
Feature's of Charcot's Joint

Grotesque deformity
Unexplained deformity with known neuropathy
Lax deformity: increased passive range of motion
Slippage when bearing weight
Lack of tenderness
Feel like "bag of bones"

Goal. *Distinguish between ankle arthritis and dependent edema.*

Technique. Check for symmetry, pitting in skin, and tenderness during passive motion.

Interpretation.

1. Both processes can fill in hollows anterior to the medial and lateral malleoli.
2. Bilaterality favors edema. Unilaterality is harder to interpret, since dependent edema may falsely localize and mimic ankle effusion.
3. Red, warm, tender pitting skin may reflect arthritis or cellulitis.
4. Tenderness is much more common with inflammation but is also found with tense edema (shows loss of skin creases and wrinkles and a shiny, atrophic look).
5. If limitation of motion exceeds that expected for the degree of swelling, ankle arthritis becomes more likely.
6. Disappearance after elevation, compression, or diuretics favors edema but does not prove it.

FEET AND TOES

Technique. A pillowcase or paper towel is placed on the ground for the patient to stand on. Inspect the patient's feet and toes from all sides, with his feet parallel to one another and bearing equal weight. Then with both of you seated, examine the patient's foot elevated onto an examining stool. Proper visualization of the sole requires that the patient lie down and that you look from the foot of table. Exposing the heel can be done as indicated in Table 10.16.

Table 10.16
Alternative Methods for Bringing the Heel Into View (in Descending Order of Patient Strength)

Have patient kneel backward on chair, hands on chair back.
Have patient lie prone and flex knee, look on from head of table.
Put patient into lateral decubitus position.

Other Foot and Toe Tests

- *Achilles tendon:* Inspect for contracture; palpate for xanthomas.
- *Ankle mortise:* Palpate with both thumbs pressing just anterior to the malleoli and with all eight fingers curled around the back of the ankle and heel.
- *Midfoot and forefoot:* Squeeze all five metatarsophalangeal joints at the base of the toes, using a single hand.
- **Diabetic foot ulcers:** Study the sole especially; if you find any sore, note the deepest tissue layer involved and measure it with a ruler in two dimensions. Record it in a sketch.
- *Toes:* Inspect the toes with the patient standing; look for dependent rubor. With the patient supine, look at and between the toes for maceration and soft corns.
- *Toenails:* At the toenails, look for
  Macerated, softened, irregular nails
  Hard, thickened, ridged, yellowed nails
  Erythema and tenderness where the lateral margin of the nail undermines the lateral nail bed, with or without expressible pus and with or without erythema and fluctuance of immediately adjacent skin
  Uniform whitening of nails
  Long recurved uncut nails
  Interpretation.
- The foot can show pressure effects such as **corns**—thickly keratinized tissue overlying the dorsum of one or more distal phalanges—and **calluses**-pads of heaped—up keratin on the soles or over the lateral protuberances of the forefoot.

  Pes planus is a very flat arch **(flatfoot)**, and pes cavus is the opposite, an unusually high instep arch. Pes cavus can come from common peroneal nerve damage. Pes equinus can result from disease or from the chronic wearing of high-heeled shoes.

  Metatarsophalangeal arthritis, with tenderness and sometimes effusion, is common in rheumatoid arthritis.

At the first metatarsophalangeal joint, consider gouty arthritis also.

Callosities under metatarsal heads suggest *(a)* intrinsic disease of foot, *(b)* abnormality of any muscle inserted in it, *(c)* abnormal stance and gait, or *(d)* effects of **ill-fitting footwear**.

The usual site attacked by both **gout** and **bunion** is the medial aspect of the first metatarsophalangeal joint. During an acute gout attack, this will be red, hot, swollen, and extraordinarily tender. The major differential diagnosis is septic arthritis. When a reddened but only mildly tender focus is found over the head of the first metatarsal, bunion is most likely.

- **Diabetic foot ulcers** become portals of entry for microbes that amplify the tissue injury. If fat, tendon, bone, or a base obscured by exudate is seen, **osteomyelitis** is likely. Unfortunately, osteomyelitis is frequent even when a diabetic foot ulcer appears shallow.

- Normal toes lie flat on the floor when bearing weight. In **hallux valgus** deformity, the great toe is laterally deviated, often leading to bunion formation medially.

The normally flat toes may become pathologically flexed at the distal interphalangeal joint, resulting in *hammertoe deformity*, most often on the second toe, which involves hyperextension of the metatarsophalangeal joint, flexion of PIP, and hyperextension of the distal interphalangeal joint.

Clawtoes usually affect all five toes on a foot and are frequently associated with pes cavus. They result from hyperextension of metatarsophalangeal joints and flexion of both interphalangeal joints of each toe. Because of abnormal weight bearing, they often lead to callosities on the plantar aspects of some metatarsal heads and of some or all toe tips and on the dorsa of affected toes.

Maceration between toes is commonly associated with superficial mycosis; the cracks can become a portal of bacterial entry.

- Nail irregularities are indicative of various conditions.

  Macerated, softened, irregular nails are often *infected* and characteristically not well cared for.

  Thick, ridged yellow nails constitute *onychauxis,* which may reflect chronic ischemia, nail dystrophy, or fungal infection.

  When *ingrowing toenails* cause inflammation of skin adjoining a toenail margin, this is **paronychia.** Erythema is expected, as is tenderness, unless neuropathy blocks it; fluctuance and expressible pus are common.

  White nails are most commonly seen in cirrhosis.

  Long uncut nails are **ram's horn nails (*ony-chogryphosis*).** Such nails can interfere with gait and with wearing of shoes. They also imply a self-care deficit that may have roots in physical disability, psychopathology, or social and financial problems.

Peripheral Nerves and Muscles

Goal. Evaluate integrity of regional neuromuscular apparatus.

Technique. To evaluate the *common peroneal* nerve, watch the gait for

1. Knees raised higher to keep the foot from scraping the floor with each step, because the foot does not dorsiflex properly
2. A foot that slaps the ground
3. Dorsiflexion by having the patient walk on his heels to see dorsiflexion ability

Interpretation. Common peroneal palsy is the usual cause of a high-knee-raising **steppage gait.** Associated inability to dorsiflex properly is highlighted by failure of attempted walking on heels with the forefoot elevated. Besides some motor tests, normal sensation in the dorsal web between the hallux and second toe—analogous to the radial nerve territory in the hand—demonstrates preserved tibial nerve function and excludes a full-blown sciatic nerve lesion.

Goal. Evaluate monoparesis or hemiparesis for psychogenic component.

Technique. When a patient attempts to raise a paralyzed limb, there is normally involuntary movement of its mate downward to gain leverage. This is the basis of *Hoover's test* for nonorganic paresis. Have the patient lie supine. Stand at the foot of the bed and cup your hands around both heels. Have the patient try to raise his weak leg off the bed. There should be marked downward pressure from involuntary hip extension pressure on the sound side.

Interpretation. *In bilateral disease the test is invalid.* In unilateral weakness, however, failure of downward pressure by the "good" heel implicates poor effort.

11

Neurologic Examination

Equipment and supplies needed for the neurologic examination are listed in Table 11.1. Begin neurologic evaluation

Table 11.1
Supplies and Equipment for the Neurologic Examination

Reflex hammer
Tuning fork, low frequency (128 Hz)
Cotton wisp or fluffed cotton swab
Pointed instrument: broken swab-stick, small key
Stethoscope
Ophthalmoscope
Snellen chart

from the first moment you meet the patient. The patient's behavior and mood during medical history taking provide clues to his neurologic and emotional state; and subsequent mental status examination is guided by observations of general appearance, affect, and cognitive interaction. Evaluate the patient's speech and hearing throughout the interview. Movements and transfers of the body during physical examination also provide important data. Check cranial nerves II–XII during the head examination, and check muscle strength, tone, and muscle-group functions during examination of the limbs. Check other components after the patient has assumed the sitting position.

INTEGRATIVE CEREBRAL FUNCTION
(INCLUDING MENTAL STATUS EXAMINATION)

Goal. Determine the patient's global brain function.

Technique. If you have been observing higher brain functions throughout the medical history taking, you will already have a sound impression about level of consciousness, speech pattern, mood and affect, concentration ability, short-term memory, and orientation. Since capable conversationalists can harbor unrecognized severe brain dysfunction when social grace is preserved, *formally* test cortical function. To screen cortical function, have the patient state his name, the date and day of the week, month, and year, and where the encounter is occurring (town, name of institution).

Memory. **Memory testing** is divided into three components:

1. *Immediate memory:*
   a. Repeat a series of three to five numbers.
   b. Repeat a series of three to five nouns, e.g., pen, tree, apple, table, house.
2. *Recent memory:*
   a. Instruct the patient to repeat and later recall a list of three objects. Go on with other parts of examination; in 2–5 minutes, have the patient recall the items.
   b. Have the patient repeat something he told you earlier in the interview.
3. *Remote memory:*
   a. Have the patient list dates of major life events such as birth of children and age of retirement.
   b. Have the patient name the United States presidents from the present backward, as far as possible.

Reasoning. Have the patient describe what he would do if he found a stamped, addressed letter lying on the sidewalk. If he says anything other than "put it in nearest mailbox," have him explain, so you can follow his **reasoning**.

Abstraction. Have the patient interpret any proverb; look for the ability to move beyond the concrete; e.g., "What does 'A stitch in time saves nine' mean?"

Folstein Mini-Mental Status Examination. The **Folstein Mini-Mental Status Examination** (Fig. 11.1) tests attention, registration, memory, and praxis.

Language and speech. Unintelligible speech may be due to motor dysfunction, hearing loss (insufficient feedback), or cerebral impairment. Dysarthria, the inability to articulate,

Mini-Mental Status Examination (MMSE)

Add points for each correct response.

		Score	Points
Orientation			
1. What is the:	Year	_____	1
	Season	_____	1
	Date	_____	1
	Day	_____	1
	Month	_____	1
2. Where are we?	Country	_____	1
	State	_____	1
	Town or city	_____	1
	Hospital	_____	1
	Floor	_____	1

Registration
3. Name three objects, taking one second to   _____   3
   say each. Then ask the patient to repeat all
   three after you have said them. Give one
   point for each correct answer. Repeat the
   answers until patient learns ✔ all three.

Attention and calculation
4. Spell WORLD backwards. One point for   _____   5
   each correct letter.

Recall
5. Ask for names of three objects learned in   _____   3
   question #3. Give one point for each correct answer.

Language
6. Point to a pen and a watch. Have the patient   _____   2
   name them as you point.
7. Have the patient repeat "No ifs, ands, or buts."   _____   1
8. Have the patient follow a three-stage command: _____   3
   "Take a paper in your right hand. Fold the paper
   in half. Put the paper on the floor."
9. Have the patient read and obey the following: _____   1
   "CLOSE YOUR EYES." (Print it in large letters.)
10. Have the patient write a sentence of his or her   _____   1
    choice. (The sentence should contain a subject
    and an object and should make sense. Ignore
    spelling errors when scoring.)
11. Have the patient copy the design. (Give one   _____   1
    point if all sides and angles are preserved and
    if the intersecting sides form a quadrangle. Use
    a large stimulus.)   _____ Total 30

Figure 11.1 Folstein Mini-Mental Status Examination form.

can occur with disease of tongue, palate, jaw, lips, pharynx; **dysphonia** is voice change, most commonly hoarseness, which occurs with vocal cord pathology. Accurate testing for ability to use **language** requires that the patient be able to hear and to comprehend instructions and, for some tests, to have sight and intact vocal apparatus.

1. *Verbal expression* (abnormality is expressive, anterior, or *Broca's aphasia*):
   a. Does the patient use enough words to make complete sentences (apart from interruptions)?
   b. Does the patient understand requests but have difficulty "getting out" or finding words of response?
   c. Does the patient invariably respond with repetitive "stock" phrases?
   d. Does the patient use incorrect word substitutes, such as "bat" for "ball" (paraphasias), or create meaningless words (neologisms)?
   e. Does the patient struggle *excessively* to find the right word, often failing altogether (anomia)?
2. *Written expression* (abnormality is *agraphia*): Can the patient write his name and address? Write a simple sentence? Copy a written sentence?
3. *Comprehension of spoken language* (abnormality is receptive, posterior, or **Wernicke's aphasia**):
   a. Can the patient pick common objects from a group: "Point to penny, point to key."
   b. Can the patient follow simple commands: "Pick up key, touch your nose with one finger."
4. *Comprehension of written language:*
   a. Give the patient written instructions: "Draw a circle on paper."
   b. Signal the patient to match *written* names of simple objects to the objects themselves (key, coin, pencil).
5. *Recognition of sense stimuli* (abnormality is *agnosia*):
   a. *Tactile:* Have the patient identify, with eyes closed, numbers drawn by a blunt object on the palm of the hand. This **graphesthesia** can be

tested only if primary sensory modalities are intact. Have the patient identify, with eyes closed, common objects placed in the hand (key, pencil, coin), i.e., **stereognosis**.

  b. *Visual:* Can the patient recognize objects and symbols by sight? Have the patient name objects as you point to them.

6. *Ability to carry out concerted, purposeful movement* (abnormality is **apraxia**):

  a. Can the patient use a pencil, key, or spoon?

  b. Have the patient walk across the room to a given destination.

Frontal lobe signs are described in Table 11.2.

Table 11.2
Frontal Lobe Signs[a]

---

1. *Glabellar:* Gently tap patient's forehead between eyebrows with your finger; normally no response or a single initial blink. Positive: exaggerated eye blinking, upper facial grimacing.
2. *Snout:* Place your finger vertically over patient's lips and tap lightly with a reflex hammer. Positive: puckering of lips.
3. *Sucking (rooting) reflex:* Lightly stimulate corners of patient's mouth with tongue blade. Positive: patient tries to grasp stimulating object with lips and to suck it.
4. *Grasp reflex:* Lightly stroke palm of patient's hand with your finger. Positive: involuntary grasp, then difficulty releasing the fingers.
5. *Palmomental reflex:* Lightly stroke palm of patient's hand. Observe patient's face for (abnormal) twitch of chin.

---

[a]Must interpret with caution.

Interpretation. Symptoms and signs of *cortical disease* concern integration and interpretation of language, memory, intellect, personality, and sensorimotor function. Impaired consciousness, intellectual or behavioral aberrations, and impairment of motor and sensory function *on both sides of the body* suggest bilateral (or diffuse) hemispheric involvement.

Anterior frontal lobe disease may impair intellectual function and personality without other neurologic signs.

Cortical localizations related to function are shown in Figure 11.2.

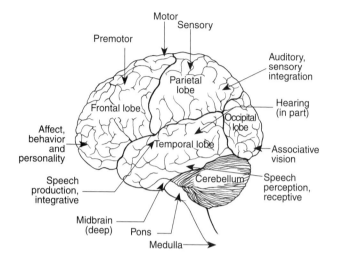

Figure 11.2 Cerebral landmarks in relation to neurologic function.

Unless psychiatrically impaired, the normal adult is appropriately dressed and groomed, interactive with your words and actions, able to carry out tasks unless non-neurologically physically impaired, and displays normal speech patterns for language background and education. Orientation to person, time, and place is accurate. We are all occasionally transiently unclear about the day of the month. Institutionalized patients may be confused as to the precise date or day of the week, although the patient should know the year and season.

The Folstein Mini-Mental Status Examination is interpreted based on score: Scores of 23 or less represent symptomatic dysfunction, and scores below 20 usually indicate psychosis, delirium, dementia, or psychotic depression. Sources of false-positive tests include inattention resulting from distraction, depression, or other psychiatric disease; sensory loss; motor impairment preventing writing or copying; linguistic difficulty; or low educational level.

Defects in various tests of language define diverse **aphasias**, apraxias, dysarthrias, and dysphonias (the last two reflect difficulty in producing the sound, not a cognitive defect).

Four abnormal levels of consciousness are described:

1. *Hypervigilant:* intensely responsive to even the lightest activity in environment
2. *Lethargic:* drowsiness, mild blunting of consciousness, slowed reactions; no spontaneous behavior
3. *Stuporous* (obtunded): severely drowsy, difficult to arouse
4. *Comatose:* no response, except reflex, to any stimulus

HEAD AND INTRACRANIAL STATUS

Goal. Determine if the patient's intracranial pressure is elevated.

Technique. Look for loss of retinal venous pulsations and for lateral rectus muscle weakness.

Interpretation. **Retinal venous pulsations** can be lost within minutes of a rise in intracranial pressure. The later ophthalmoscopic signs of **papilledema** may be delayed 24 hours after pressure rises and may persist 24 hours after it falls. Pulsations clearly indicate no elevated pressure, but *the absence of pulsations may be normal in some individuals.* Bilateral weakness of lateral gaze (cranial nerve VI palsy) *can* be an early sign of increased intracranial pressure.

MENINGES

Goal. Look for signs of meningeal irritation.

Technique and interpretation. See Table 11.3.

CRANIAL NERVE EVALUATION

Goal. Seek disorder of peripheral portions of these nerves or their representation in brainstem or cortex, which encompasses some special sensory testing.

Technique. Described with head (Chapter 4) and neck (Chapter 5).

Interpretation. Because of dense packing of sensory and motor tracts that traverse the brainstem region, even small lesions can produce multiple functional deficits.

Table 11.3
Meningeal Irritation Signs

a. *Brudzinski's nape of neck sign:* With patient supine, passively flex patient's neck toward chest, cradling occiput in your hands. Resistance to flexion is **meningismus**; involuntary flexion of hips and knees is a positive Brudzinski's nape of neck sign.
b. *Brudzinski's contralateral reflex signs:* Identical contralateral reflex sign is elicited when you passively flex patient's hip and knee on one side and contralateral leg begins to flex. If one leg flexes on passive flexion of other leg and then extends spontaneously, *reciprocal* contralateral reflex has occurred.
c. *Straight-leg-raising (Lasègue) test:* With patient supine, flex patient's thigh by lifting leg by heel, keeping knee extended. Positive: limitation of hip flexion by pain and/or hamstring muscle spasm. In contrast to positive unilateral straight-leg raising found in localized lumbosacral nerve root irritation, *meningeal irritation response is bilateral.*
d. *Kernig's sign:* With patient supine, passively flex patient's hip and knee together; then sharply extend patient's knee by raising heel and knee together. Positive: spasm (not pain) prevents full extension of knee.

Regarding visual field cuts, most of the visual radiations lie in the temporal lobes, such that homonymous hemianopia or quadrantanopsia indicates a brain lesion contralateral to the field loss, e.g., *left* temporal lobe with *right* homonymous hemianopsia. Occipital lobe disease is suggested by contralateral **homonymous hemianopsia,** visual agnosia, and loss of reading comprehension.

SPINAL CORD, NERVE ROOT AND PERIPHERAL NERVE FUNCTION

Goal. Determine integrity of the regional apparatus from cervical cord through cauda equina.

Technique. Study sensory, motor, and reflex functions as listed below.

Interpretation. Relevant spinal cord and root anatomy is shown in Figure 11.3.

1. Regardless of axial location, a *lesion of the spinal cord,* whether intrinsic or externally compressive, will eventually produce both segmental signs (lower motor neuron signs, dermatomal sensory loss, and

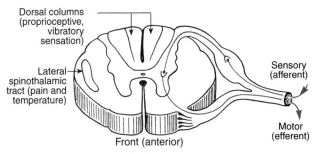

Figure 11.3 Cross-section of spinal cord and nerve root.

local reflex depression or loss) and long tract signs, both sensory and motor.

2. *Cauda equina syndrome* causes lower motor neuron paralysis involving both thigh and leg, often asymmetrical, associated with reduction of patellar and Achilles reflexes, dermatomal sensory loss below the upper lumbar segments, and bladder and rectal dysfunction. Pain is usually prominent, as may be saddle-area hypesthesia.

3. *Classic nerve root problems* are indicated by weakness, pain, sensory loss, and reflex depression exclusively in the distribution of affected nerve(s).

4. *Plexus* or multiple nerve root lesions show symptoms and signs that extend over multiple nerve root distributions.

5. *Mononeuropathy* indicates that a single nerve is involved, most often from compression, e.g., entrapment.

6. *Peripheral neuropathy* is indicated by weakness, decreased stretch reflexes, and decreased sensation most typically in a stocking or a glove-and-stocking pattern. Usually symmetrical widespread dysfunction, often worse in the lower limbs.

7. *Muscle weakness without sensory loss* may be *either neuronal or myopathic*. Muscle stretch reflexes are diminished or lost when nerve is involved but are preserved longer when the problem arises in muscle.

Muscle fasciculation suggests a neural rather than a primary muscular disorder.

SENSORY EVALUATION

Goal. Study the afferent function of peripheral nerves, roots, and spinal cord, including separating out **posterior column function**.

Technique. Consider superficial pain and touch, vibration, and joint position sense. Successful sensory examination requires full concentration, comprehension of task, and cooperation from the patient. Perform all maneuvers with the patient's eyes closed or averted to avoid visual cuing.

1. *Light touch:* Use fingertip or cotton wisp. Say, "Tell me each time you feel this and where. Please close your eyes."

2. *Superficial pain:* Try a broken tongue blade alternating with an intact one. Say, "Tell me each time whether you feel sharp or dull."

3. *Joint position sense:* If toe joint position sense is intact, proximal position sense is assumed to be normal. Tell the patient, "I will be moving your toe; each time I move it, tell me whether it has moved toward the floor or the ceiling." Test the metatarsophalangeal joint of each great toe. Grasp the digit distal to the joint *firmly* by its upper and lower surfaces and move it through a range up and down.

4. *Vibratory sense:* Place the stem of a vibrating low-frequency tuning fork (128 Hz) against a bony prominence, typically the medial malleolus, and say, "Please describe what you feel, where you feel it, and when it stops." If the patient perceives *vibration* and not merely touch, when the patient says vibrations have stopped, touch the stem of the fork to a comparable site on your own body. Cease at the periphery if normal.

5. *Sensory deficits:* To map sensory deficits, move the stimulus from hypesthesia to its margins, drawing with a skin pencil the boundaries of loss. Proximal testing of vibration or position moves from ankle to

shin to femoral condyle to iliac crest until a zone
with normal vibratory sense has been found.

   Pressure on the sternum is the standard method in
the comatose patient.

6. *Temperature perception* (checked if superficial pain
   is absent in a limb): Ask the patient to discriminate,
   with eyes closed, between a warm test tube of water
   and a cold one or between any two objects of similar
   texture but different temperatures.

7. *Bilateral simultaneous stimulation:* First ask the
   patient to indicate where he (with eyes closed) feels
   stimulus as a finger is touched to each limb in turn;
   if he can perceive and localize a single stimulus
   accurately at each site, then apply two equal stimuli
   simultaneously to symmetrical body areas, and ask
   the same question again to determine whether he
   perceives both stimuli at once. Abnormalities reflect
   defective cortical integration, typically in the
   parietal lobes.

8. *Romberg test:* This test further assesses posterior
   column function. Have the patient stand erect, with
   feet together and arms extended forward, first with
   eyes open and then with eyes closed. Stand near
   enough to catch the patient and prevent a fall if the
   patient loses his balance. If the patient loses his balance and sways dangerously with eyes open, do not
   proceed to the second step.

Interpretation. Figure 11.4, *A* and *B,* shows dermatomal
sensory function, while Figure 11.5, *A* and *B,* shows sensory
peripheral nerves. Inferences about sensory loss *patterns* are
in Table 11.4.

Discrimination between "sharp" and "dull" depends on
clarity of stimuli. Calloused soles have sensory endings
entombed in keratin and thus protected from sensation;
they ought not be tested for light touch or superficial pain.

If you feel continuing vibration from the tuning fork
after the patient does not, the patient has impaired vibratory
sensation. Joint position sense does *not* suffer age-related

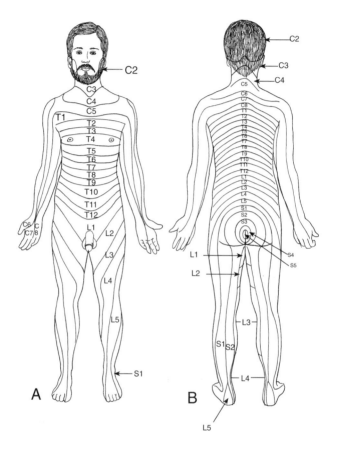

Figure 11.4 Dermatomes. **A.** Anterior view. **B.** Posterior view.

decline; thus, test this modality, instead of vibration, in aged persons to study the posterior columns of the cord.

If the patient identifies each individual stimulus correctly but loses one side on bilateral simultaneous stimulation, **extinction** characteristic of nondominant parietal lobe disease is indicated

Unless there is a structural musculoskeletal problem, a neurologically intact person can stand in the Romberg posi-

Table 11.4
Common Sensory Loss Patterns

Site of Lesion	Distribution of Sensory Loss
Cerebral hemisphere	Contralateral face and body: loss of discrimination and/or integration
Brainstem	Ipsilateral face/contralateral body: loss of pain and temperature
Transverse section of spinal cord, complete	Below level of lesion: bilateral loss all sensory modalities
Hemitransection of spinal cord (Brown-Séquard syndrome)	Below level of lesion: ipsilateral loss of position sense and vibration, contralateral loss of pain and temperature
Posterior columns of spinal cord	Below level of lesion: bilateral loss or attenuation of position sense (proprioception) and vibration
Spinal nerve roots	Variable, may have none at all (see Fig. 11.4)
Polyneuropathy	Varying degrees of loss in glove-and-stocking distribution, gradually improving from distal to proximal
Major peripheral nerves	See Fig. 11.5

tion with eyes closed for 15 seconds without falling, retropulsion, or significant swaying.

MOTOR EVALUATION

Goal. Determine adequacy of the corticospinal tract-nerve-muscle unit for mobilizing body parts and supporting somatic function.

Technique. Assess the strength of muscle groups by resistance testing. In seeking subtle hemiparesis, seek the *digiti quinti sign*; i.e., have the patient extend his arms, palms down and fingers pressed initially into adduction by you; look for abduction of the affected fifth finger only.

Define **distribution** of any **weakness**. Is it served by the motor cortex above the pyramidal decussation? by long tracts below the pyramidal decussation but above the thoracic cord such that the face is spared from paresis? by corticospinal tract(s) in or below the thoracic cord such that the face *and arms* are spared? by a single or several adjacent spinal segments, unilateral or bilateral? by a peripheral nerve?

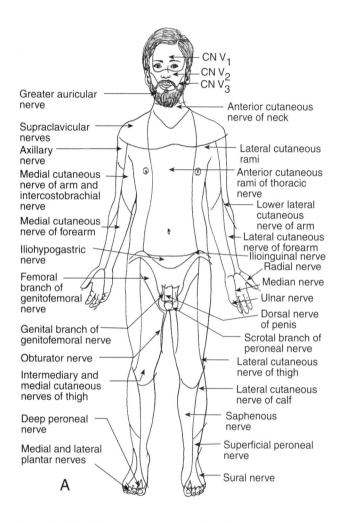

Figure 11.5 Peripheral nerve representations in cutaneous innervation. **A.** Anterior view. **B.** Posterior view.

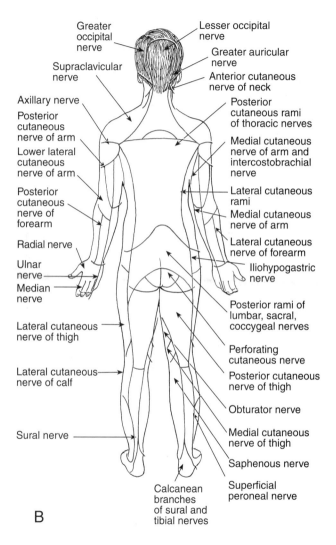

Greater occipital nerve
Lesser occipital nerve
Greater auricular nerve
Supraclavicular nerve
Anterior cutaneous nerve of neck
Axillary nerve
Posterior cutaneous nerve of arm
Lower lateral cutaneous nerve of arm
Posterior cutaneous nerve of forearm
Radial nerve
Ulnar nerve
Median nerve
Lateral cutaneous nerve of thigh
Lateral cutaneous nerve of calf
Sural nerve
Posterior cutaneous rami of thoracic nerves
Medial cutaneous nerve of arm and intercostobrachial nerve
Lateral cutaneous rami
Medial cutaneous nerve of arm
Lateral cutaneous nerve of forearm
Iliohypogastric nerve
Posterior rami of lumbar, sacral, coccygeal nerves
Perforating cutaneous nerve
Posterior cutaneous nerve of thigh
Obturator nerve
Medial cutaneous nerve of thigh
Saphenous nerve
Superficial peroneal nerve
Calcanean branches of sural and tibial nerves

B

Figure 11.5 **B.**

Define **degree** of weakness as in Table 11.5. Also, seek **atrophy**—decreased muscle mass—in the area under ques-

Table 11.5
Muscle Group Strength

Score	Interpretation
5	Normal
4	Overcome by examiner's resistance more readily than average normal control patients (note that this definition allows for the large range of strength of examiners)
3	Can move against gravity but not with added examiner resistance
2	Can move only if gravity is eliminated, I.e., sideways or on a surface
1	Only a trace of contraction
0	No muscular contraction

tion. Define tone by passive movement of joints served by muscles being evaluated and by palpation. Are muscles lax (flaccid) or rigid (spastic)? tender? Seek absent or decreased resistance to passive movement (atonia or hypotonia) and increased resistance (spasticity). If spasticity is noted on initial rapid extension but disappears as extension is continued, the "clasp-knife phenomenon" is indicated. A repeated ratcheting, catch-release response as you extend the joint (cogwheel rigidity) is characteristic of disease of the basal nuclei.

Observe muscles for **abnormal involuntary movements** such as fasciculations (fine, random spontaneous twitches visible at skin surface over muscle) and the more regular small movements of **tremor.** Of particular importance in persons taking neuroleptic drugs is assessment for tardive dyskinesias. In assessing involuntary movements, observe
1. *Tremor* for
    a. Precise location (fingers, arms, legs, etc.)
    b. Laterality (unilateral, symmetric, or asymmetric)
    c. Quality (fine or coarse, rhythmic or erratic)
    d. Effect of *purposeful* movement, i.e., tremor present only at rest (resting tremor), exacerbated by purposeful movement such as reaching for something (intention tremor), present only when

       muscles are stretched and extended as with
       spreading fingers (postural tremor)

2. *Chorea*, rapid, jerky, purposeless contractions of random muscle groups
3. *Athetosis*, slow, writhing irregular movements that begin randomly in one muscle group and spread to adjoining groups
4. *Dystonia*, parts of body held in abnormal postures for longer periods of time than observed in ordinary daily life
5. *Hemiballism*, abrupt, unilateral violent flinging at proximal joints
6. *Tic*, spastic twitching of small muscle groups, often on the face
7. *Asterixis* (see Chapter 10, Limbs)

Interpretation. See Table 11.5 for grading of muscular strength.

The *digiti quinti sign*, whereby the fifth finger on the affected limb is abducted while the pinkie finger on the normal side remains adducted, indicates mild hemiparesis.

Upper motor neuron (UMN) lesions may lie in the cerebral cortex, corticobulbar tracts, or corticospinal tracts; lower motor neuron (LMN) lesions involve anterior horn cells or their axons. UMN lesions typically cause relatively few of the same signs as LMN lesions. Table 11.6 contrasts their features.

Table 11.6
Signs of Upper Versus Lower Motor Neuron Disease

	Upper Motor Neuron	Lower Motor Neuron
Tone	Spastic,[a] greater in flexors of arms, extensors of legs	Flaccid
Reflexes	Accentuated stretch reflexes[a]	Normal, decreased, or absent
Babinski	Present	Absent
Clonus	Frequently present	Absent
Muscle bulk	Slightly atrophy of disuse only, late	Atrophy, often marked
Fasciculations	No	Yes

[a] Note that very shortly after an injury to the brain or spinal cord, upper motor neuron signs may be lacking, and there may even be falsely localizing lower motor neuron signs. This transient state is known as **cerebral shock** or **spinal shock,** respectively, notwithstanding that it produces no hypotension.

Most involuntary movements reflect disease of the **extrapyramidal** system, with limb movements occurring contralateral to the brain lesion. Other signs that can arise in this system are muscle rigidity and slowness of movement (bradykinesia). The combination of hypotonia, difficulty in performing tests of coordination, and imbalance of stance or a wide-based gait even with eyes open suggests **cerebellar disease.** The combination of lack of coordination and abnormal stance with eyes closed that improves when the patient watches his movements suggests **proprioceptive dysfunction,** although cerebellar dysfunction with visual compensation is an alternative explanation. Cogwheel rigidity, a shuffling gait with knees and arms slightly flexed, armswing diminution or loss, and festinating gait wherein the patient's legs seem to be trying to catch up with his trunk are typical of **parkinsonism.**

Gait

Goals. Rapidly assess global motor function; determine a vital outcome of having satisfactory motor function and integration, i.e., producing a function essential for usual active living.

Technique. For patients who are not bed- or wheelchair-bound, observation of **gait** is the highest-yield component of the neurologic examination. Employ cane, walker, crutches, or assistants for support. Feet should be bare or stockinged. Observe for smoothness of gait, placement of feet (broad-based or normal), symmetry of leg and arm movement, step height (normal or shuffling), step length (normal or shortened), staggering, or uncertainty. Then have the patient turn around, and note the number of steps required to achieve this. Additional useful maneuvers, if there is suspicion of a gait abnormality, include tandem walking (heel to toe, Fig. 11.6*A*), hopping on one foot at a time, walking on toes (Fig. 11.6*B*) and then on heels (Fig. 11.6*C*), and the Tinetti mobility test (Chapter 10).

Interpretation. Normal gait—including the stressful subvariants—implies considerable but not necessarily perfect integrity of lower limb strength, proprioception, cere-

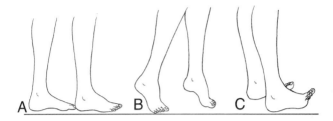

Figure 11.6 Gait evaluation. **A.** Tandem gait. **B.** Walking on toes. **C.** Walking on heels.

bellar coordination, and cortical integration. With aging, gait slows and becomes somewhat hesitant.

REFLEXES

Muscle Stretch Reflexes

Goal. Assess function of reflex arcs with special attention given to effects of disinhibition from above or intrinsic cord disease.

Technique. Elicitation of a stretch reflex requires a relaxed muscle group, aversion of the patient's gaze to avoid anticipatory muscle tensing, accurate localization of the tendon to be tapped, and a loose, swinging motion of the hammer from your wrist to facilitate sudden displacement.

If you are having trouble getting a lower limb reflex, ask the patient to place his hands in position to tug at one another on command (Fig. 11.7), raise his eyes toward the ceiling, and await your verbal command to "pull." With patient thus positioned in readiness, have him pull while you *immediately* strike the tendon and observe for muscle contraction. This **Jendrassik maneuver** can bring out latent reflexes. For reinforcement of upper limb reflexes, the patient clenches his teeth (to create an arc above the cervical cord).

For **triceps reflex testing**, place the patient's upper arm in the palm of your hand such that his forearm swings loosely with the elbow bent and upper arm *hyper*adducted onto the thorax. Find the triceps tendon as it attaches to the olecranon on the extensor surface of the distal arm; strike

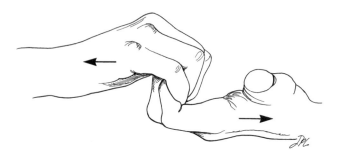

Figure 11.7 Reinforcement of reflexes with hand tugging (Jendrassik maneuver).

the tendon sharply with the broad side of the reflex hammer. Observe for contraction of the triceps muscle, which will tend to extend the elbow.

For **biceps reflex testing**, have the patient rest his arm in his lap, which will force it into moderate flexion at the elbow. Place the thumb of your nondominant hand over the biceps tendon while curling other fingers around the distal upper arm. Strike your thumb with the point of the hammer, transmitting a stimulus to the tendon. Observe the biceps for contraction, which further flexes the forearm.

For **brachioradialis reflex**, with the patient's arm resting in his lap, locate the brachioradialis muscle on the radial surface of the mid to upper forearm; and strike the tendon lightly. Look for radial deviation of the wrist and thumb or extension of the wrist, index finger, or middle finger.

For **patellar reflex testing**, have the patient sit with legs dangling free. Locate the tendon just distal to the patella; strike the tendon once, observing for quadriceps contraction and/or resultant extension of the knee.

The **Achilles reflex** is toughest to elicit correctly. With the patient's feet free, find the Achilles tendon and place the palm of your nondominant hand on the sole of the patient's foot, applying *slight* upward pressure. Tap the tendon briskly with the broad base of the hammer. Observe for plantar flexion; i.e., a *push* of the forefoot against your palm. If this is not elicited, have the patient kneel on a chair seat, with his feet hanging free over the edge of the seat, and repeat the maneuvers with free view of the tendon (Fig. 11.8). To reinforce in this position, have the patient grip the chair back as you strike the tendon—a perfect Jendrassik equivalent.

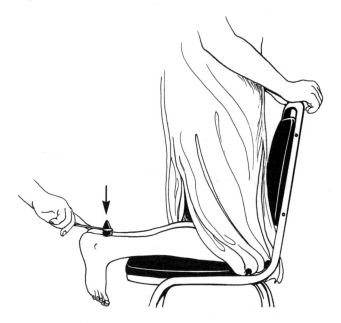

Figure 11.8 Achilles (ankle) reflex with patient kneeling.

Interpretation. Symmetry of response is essential in stretch reflexes, the levels of representation of which are given in Table 11.7; the range of responses is listed in Table 11.8. An occasional healthy adult will have absent paired reflexes. A significant minority of elderly patients lose reflexes at the ankles. Thus, normal individuals may have responses of 0, 1, or 2. The only grades that are *always* abnormal are 3 and 4; others are suspect if altered over time, if discordant with other findings, or if asymmetric.

Table 11.7
Levels of Common Reflexes[a]

Muscle stretch reflexes
       Biceps brachii reflex: *C5*, C6
       Brachioradialis reflex: C5, *C6*
       Triceps brachii reflex: C6, *C7*, C8
       Patellar reflex (knee jerk): L2, L3, *L4*
       Achilles reflex (ankle jerk): *S1*, S2
Superficial reflexes
       Plantar response: L4, L5, *S1*, S2
       Abdominal upper quadrants: T7–T9
       Abdominal lower quadrants: T11–L1
       Cremasteric: L1-L2

[a]Root is dominant contributor when there is one.

Table 11.8
Range of Stretch Reflex Responses

Grade	Response
0	No response elicited, with reinforcing maneuvers
+1	Response *only* with reinforcement (Jendrassik or other)
+2	Moderate response without reinforcement
+3	Brisk response, with 1–3 beats of clonus (brief terminal jerking of the muscle following the initial response)
+4	Exaggerated response with sustained clonus

Superficial Reflexes

Goal. Assay for level of spinal cord dysfunction.

Technique. Plantar response, the most important, is assessed as follows.

With a swab-stick, stroke the sole on its lateral aspect, beginning near the heel and crossing the ball of the foot to the base of the great toe. The motion is firm and continuous, noxious but neither painful nor ticklish. Observe response of the toes: Do they curl under, dorsiflex, or fan out? Alternatives to this test are given in Table 11.9.

Other superficial reflexes. Other superficial reflexes help establish a spinal cord level or a subtle unilateral lesion (see Table 11.7).

    1. *Abdominal:* With patient supine, stroke the four quadrants of the abdominal skin. Observe

Table 11.9
Alternative Reflexes to Plantar Stroking[a]

a. *Chaddock:* Stimulate superolateral aspect of patient's foot with blunt point in arc from malleolus toward base of hallux.

b. *Oppenheim's:* Apply pressure with your thumb and index finger over anterior surface of patient's tibia in downward sweep from infrapatellar region to foot.

c. *Gordon:* On deep pressure to calf muscle, look for dorsiflexion of hallux and fanning of other toes with corticospinal tract disease.

d. *Schäfer's:* On deep pressure to Achilles tendon, look for dorsiflexion response with corticospinal tract disease.

[a]None is as reliable as Babinski's reflex.

movement of the umbilicus in response. Normally, it is pulled slightly toward the quadrant being stimulated.

2. *Cremasteric:* With the patient supine and thighs slightly spread, lightly stroke the proximal inner thigh. Normally, the scrotum or labium on the stimulated side contracts cephalad.

Interpretation. The initial movement on plantar stroking is critical. Normal persons plantarflex the hallux. To dorsiflex the great toe or flare all toes is the **Babinski response**, a term applied *only* to the abnormal; a Babinski response in any person beyond the age of myelination is pathologic. Elderly patients sometimes have no plantar response; this is uninterpretable. *Bilateral* upgoing toes imply bilateral dysfunction or diffuse cerebral dysfunction.

CEREBELLAR TESTING

Goal. Determine integrative function and its effect on the smoothness of motor responses.

Technique. Performing accurate and symmetrical rapid movements requires motor control, proprioceptive joint position sense, vestibular apparatus, and cerebellar mediation.

Upper limb testing.

1. Have the patient sequentially touch the tip of each finger with the thumb of the same hand, speeding up as much as possible; test both hands simultaneously; *or*

2. Have the patient slap the backs and then the palms of both hands against his knees, progressively picking up speed; *or*
3. Have the patient touch his nose with the tip of his index finger, then extend that finger to touch your fingertip, and continue that motion back and forth between his nose and your moving finger. Observe for accuracy, speed, and symmetry as you test each side.

Lower limb testing. Have the patient perform the heel-to-shin maneuver. Say, "Place the heel of your right foot just below your left knee. Then slide it straight down your shin to your ankle and back up again as quickly and accurately as you can." Have him repeat the maneuver contralaterally. Observe for accuracy of heel placement, and note if the heel moves readily without wavering.

Interpretation. Joint or primary muscular disease may affect these maneuvers, and the aged patient may perform them more slowly, especially in the nondominant hand, but still with accuracy. "Overshooting" on the finger-to-nose tests and equivalents is *past-pointing*, a sign of cerebellar dysfunction. Poor performance, especially on the heel-to-shin maneuver, may reflect joint disease or a musculoskeletal problem, so interpret it carefully.

Three **cerebellar dysfunction** patterns are

1. Dysfunction on the ipsilateral side of the body (cortical fibers have already crossed the midline when they reach the cerebellum) characterizes a unilateral cerebellar hemispheric lesion. Muscle hypotonia, loss of coordination, and ataxia with falling *toward* the abnormal side all accord with cerebellar hemisphere disease.
2. Wide-based gait ataxia, falling to both sides, and *truncal ataxia* characterize lesions of the vermis.
3. Diffuse cerebellar disease leads to generalized ataxia (limb and trunk), speech ataxia, and bilateral nystagmus, often vertical or rotatory.

12

Lower Back

The screening lower back examination is done with the patient standing, the posterior trunk and legs fully exposed, and the feet bare. Specially indicated extensions of the examination may necessitate several changes in patient position.

INSPECTION AND PALPATION

Technique.

1. Face the patient's back to observe alignment of spine, scapulae, iliac crests, and gluteal folds. Look for a transverse crease in the skin of the lower flanks at or above the posterior superior iliac spine.
2. Face the patient's side to assess curves.
3. Palpate the lumbar and sacral spine for tenderness and the paraspinal muscles for tenderness or spasm.
4. With your palms on the patient's posterior iliac crests, place your thumbs over dimples that mark the sites of the sacroiliac joints. Assess the joints for tenderness or swelling by pressing firmly.

Interpretation.

1. Normal back alignment (Fig. 12.1A):
   a. If there is a lateral midspinal curve (scoliosis), have the patient flex forward. A **postural scoliosis** will disappear completely.
   b. Measure leg lengths. With the patient supine and legs spread slightly, stretch a cloth tape from just beneath the anterior superior iliac crest along the length of the leg, crossing medially near the knee, and bring it to the inferior margin of the medial malleolus. Record the length. Repeat this procedure for the other leg.

      Any difference > 1 cm could contribute to pelvic tilt and subsequent scoliosis. Test this

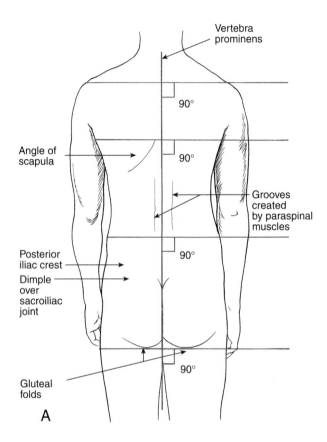

Figure 12.1 **A.** Posterior skin landmarks are superimposed on the normal back with indication of the perpendicular (right) angles that should coincide with the alignment of the spine. **B.** Lateral view showing the expected curvatures of each portion of the normal vertebral column.

contribution by placing the sole of the foot of the shorter leg on a measured lift (pad of paper) and reassess for scoliosis or tilt. If corrected by this means, the scoliosis is a **compensatory scoliosis**.

2. Normal spinal curvatures from the side (Fig. 12.1*B*): Look for abnormalities:

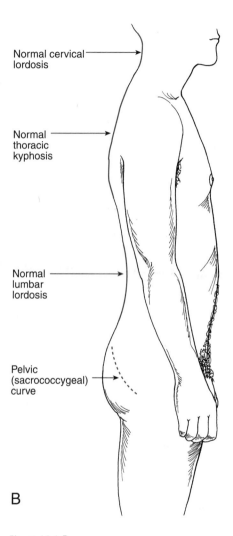

Normal cervical lordosis

Normal thoracic kyphosis

Normal lumbar lordosis

Pelvic (sacrococcygeal) curve

B

Figure 12.1 **B.**

     a. Dorsal kyphosis (see Chapter 7, Thorax and Lungs).

     b. Exaggerated lumbar lordosis: obesity, pregnancy, racial variation.

     c. Flattened lumbar curve: paraspinal muscle spasm; disease of vertebral articulations.

3. Localized vertebral tenderness: See Chapter 7, Thorax and Lungs.

4. Paraspinal muscle tenderness or spasm: Evaluate further.

5. Sacroiliac joint tenderness or swelling: Assess for other signs of inflammatory joint disease, i.e., rheumatoid arthritis or ankylosing spondylitis.

SPINAL RANGE OF MOTION

Technique. *Flexion.* Ask the patient to bend forward maximally. From behind the patient, observe movement of the spine, symmetry of the scapulae, and curvature of the flexed spine.

Extension. Ask the patient to bend backward at the waist. Observe the degree of extension achieved.

Lateral motion. Ask the patient to bend at the waist, without rotation, to each side. Assess lateral flexion for degree and symmetry.

Rotation. With your hands on the patient's iliac crests to fix the pelvis, ask the patient to rotate his upper body to one side and then to the other. Note the degree of rotation.

Interpretation. Any significant (greater than 20%) reduction in normal ranges of motion (Fig. 12.2) or any pain on motion calls for further evaluation.

HIP EXTENSION

Goal. Assess hip mobility in extension (Fig. 12.3).

Technique. Ask the patient to hyperextend each leg posteriorly while supporting himself at the end of the examining table; or, have the patient bend over the end of the table and raise each leg backward as far as it will extend.

Interpretation. See Chapter 10, Limbs.

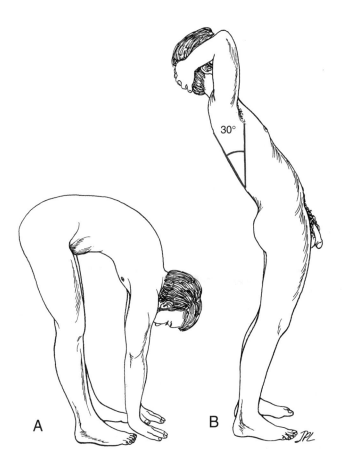

Figure 12.2 Range of motion of the spine. **A.** Full flexion with knees straight should allow the patient to place his fingertips flat on the floor. **B.** Extension approximates 30° to the vertical.

BACK PAIN EVALUATION

Goal. Evaluate complaints of back pain, pain in the leg, or limitation of motion of the back, using one or more of the following focused physical examination maneuvers (Table 12.1).

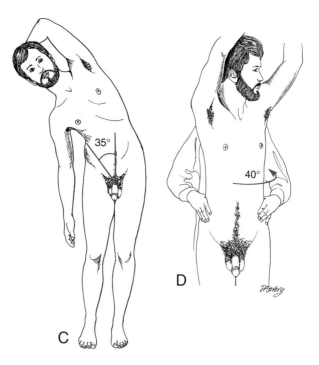

Figure 12.2—continued **C.** Lateral bending normally reaches 35° to the vertical. **D.** Rotation to right and left at 35–40°.

Schober's Flexion Test (Fig. 12.4)

Technique. With the patient standing, mark the skin over the vertebral column at the level of posterior iliac spines. Make a second mark 10 cm above the first. As the patient bends forward to touch the floor, measure the new distance between the two marks.

Interpretation. In young adults, an increase of +4 cm in the distance indicates impaired flexion. Consider spondyloarthropathy and inflammation of the paraspinous tissue.

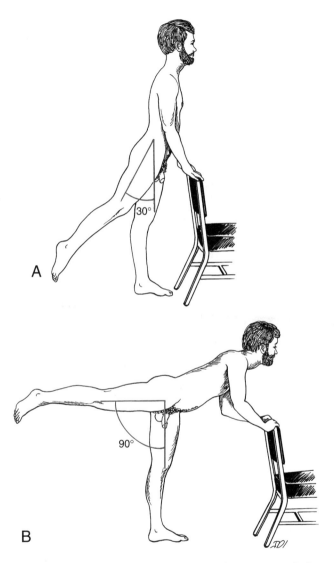

A

B

Figure 12.3 Range of hip extension. **A.** Lateral inspection with the patient standing on one leg and extending hip as far as possible. Expect 30° from the vertical. **B.** Patient supporting himself to achieve maximal hyperextension of the hip to 90° to the vertical, although no hyperextension relative to the trunk!

Table 12.1
Summary of Extended Maneuvers

Patient standing
  Inspection
    For lateral curvature
    For list
    For transverse crease
    For gap in spinous processes
    Schober's flexion test
  Palpation
    For gap in dorsal spinous processes
    For localized spinal tenderness
    For localized paraspinal muscle tenderness
    For tenderness or leg pain reproduction at sciatic notch
Patient supine
    Observe for position of maximal comfort
    Straight-leg-raising test
    Crossed straight-leg-raising test
    Foot dorsiflexion test
    Sensory examination of anterior aspects of legs and thighs
Patient prone
    Reverse straight-leg-raising test
    Sensory examination of posterior aspect of legs and thighs
Patient sitting
    Patellar (knee) and Achilles (ankle) reflexes
    Muscle group strength
Other special maneuvers when indicated
    Measurement of chest expansion
    Measurement of leg length
    Stoop test
    Tests when lack of cooperation is suspected
      Aird's test
      Bench test

Palpation With the Patient Standing

Technique. **Palpate** spinous processes for a **gap**. Palpate for **localized** spinal or paraspinal **tenderness**. If a painful site is noted, mark it with a pencil, and return later to confirm point tenderness. **Palpate the sciatic notch** and inquire about *(a)* pain radiating down one leg or the other, *(b)* an increase in preexisting pain, or *(c)* a reproduction of pain in the radiation previously described.

Interpretation. Any of the above findings suggests nerve root irritation.

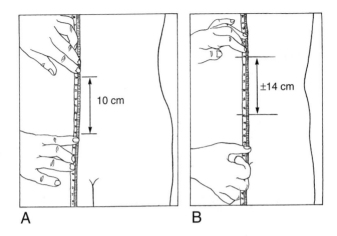

Figure 12.4 Special maneuvers. **A** and **B.** Schober's test for impaired spinal flexion. With the patient standing, a distance of 10 cm is marked off with a skin pencil **(A)**. On maximal spinal flexion, the increase in distance between the skin marks should reach or exceed 14 cm **(B)**.

Examination With the Patient Supine

Technique.
1. *Straight-leg raising:* With the patient supine, passively lift each of his extended legs in turn, noting the angle from the examining table at which the patient complains of pain in the back or down the lifted leg.
2. *Crossed straight-leg raising:* Ask the patient to raise his leg on the pain-free side to 90°. Note any complaint of exacerbated pain in the affected limb or in the previously unaffected limb.
3. *Foot dorsiflexion:* With the patient's legs on the table, sharply passively dorsiflex each of his ankles in turn.
4. *Sensory examination:* See Chapter 11, Neurologic Examination.

Interpretation.
1. Inability to raise leg to 90° without pain suggests nerve root or sciatic irritation.

Table 12.2
Possible Neurologic Abnormalities[a]

Muscles of joint motion

Joint	Motion	Nerve Root Involved if Impaired
Knee	Extension	L2–L4
	Flexion	L4–S3
Ankle	Dorsiflexion	L4–S1
	Plantar flexion	L5–S2
Foot	Supination and pronation	L4–S1
Toes	Plantar flexion	L5–S2
	Dorsiflexion	L4–S1

Loss of cutaneous sensitivity to pain (see also Chapter 11)

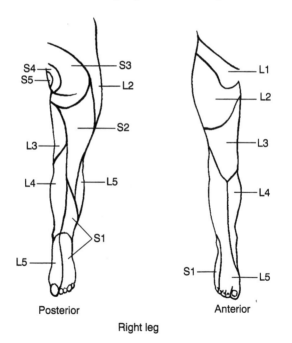

Posterior   Anterior

Right leg

[a]Lesions of single roots may produce *no* sensory deficit as a result of over-lap of innervation

2. Complaint of exacerbated pain in the affected limb or in the previously unaffected limb indicates nerve root or sciatic irritation.
3. Complaint of back pain or of pain radiating down the leg on the affected side demonstrates nerve root or sciatic nerve irritation.

Examination With the Patient Prone

Technique.
1. *Reverse straight-leg raising:* Ask the patient to flex his knee maximally.
2. *Sensory examination:* See Chapter 11, Neurologic Examination.

Interpretation. A complaint of pain in the back or in the sciatic nerve distribution on the affected side constitutes a positive test.

Examination With the Patient Sitting

Technique.
1. *Patellar and Achilles reflexes:* See Chapter 11, Neurologic Examination.
2. *Muscle group strength:* See Table 12.2 and Chapter 10, Limbs.

Interpretation. For interpretation of these results, see Chapters 10, Limbs, and 11, Neurologic Examination.

Other Special Maneuvers

STOOP TEST FOR ENTRAPMENT RADICULOPATHY

Goal. Assess for cause of intermittent, exercise-related back, gluteal, or posterior thigh pain when maneuvers outlined above fail to yield an answer.

Technique. Ask the patient to walk briskly down a corridor. Observe for progressively stooping posture.

Interpretation. A positive test consists of assuming a stooping to simian posture as walking continues and suggests entrapment such as with spinal stenosis.

TESTS FOR MALINGERING

Goal. Assess the potentially noncooperative or malingering patient.

Technique.

1. *Aird's test:* Ask the patient who could not touch his toes in standing position to do so while sitting with his supported legs extended in front of him.
2. *Bench test:* Ask the patient to kneel on a bench with hips and knees flexed and then to place his hands on the floor.

Interpretation.

1. The ability to complete this maneuver after being unable to touch toes while standing suggests a cooperation problem.
2. The patient with organic low back pain will be able to carry out this maneuver; complaint of the *inability* to do this because of pain suggests a nonorganic basis for the symptom.

COMMON CLUSTERS AND THEIR INTERPRETATIONS

Herniated Intervertebral Disc or Disc Fragments

- *Lateral deviation* toward the affected side, which persists with spinal flexion
- *Limitation of flexion and extension,* with lateral and rotational motion relatively normal
- *Paraspinal tenderness* and *muscle spasm* lateral to the spine, especially on the affected side
- *Positive straight-leg raising* with pain at <50° on the affected side
- Increased pain in the back and/or sciatic region with *crossed straight-leg raising* on the affected side and complaint of sciatic pain in the opposite leg
- Increased pain in the back and/or sciatic nerve distribution with sharp *dorsiflexion* of the foot on the affected side
- Pain in the back and/or sciatic nerve distribution on the affected side during *reverse straight-leg raising*

Lumbosacral Strain

- Accentuation of pain with spinal *flexion*.
- Accentuation of *lumbar lordosis*.
- *Spasm of paraspinal muscles* on affected side. Ask the patient to assume the position most comfortable for him, and he will usually prefer to flex his hips and knees or curl up in flexion.
- *Straight-leg raising, crossed straight-leg raising, and foot dorsiflexion* typically will not accentuate pain.
- *Neurologic* examination should be normal.

Ankylosing Spondylitis

- *Flattening of the lumbar curve*, early, progressing to rod-like spine with *forward thrust of the head*
- Tenderness on palpation of the *sacroiliac* joint
- Impairment of all ranges of *spinal motion*
- *Chest expansion* often reduced to <2 cm
- Positive *Patrick's test* (see Chapter 10, Limbs)

Spondylolisthesis

- Low back pain *referred to lateral leg or coccyx*
- *Transverse crease* of skin at or above iliac crests
- Palpable *gap* between spinous processes when anterior slippage has occurred (variable)

Osteoarthrosis of the Lower Spine

- *Pain*, when present, is low-grade and remitting.
- Patient may have *limitation of spinal motion* in any plane.
- Patient may have features of *nerve root irritation* due to osteophyte impingement.

Osteoporosis of the Spine

- Chronic *middorsal back pain*
- *Progressive loss of stature*
- Increasing *kyphosis*
- *Acute, severe pain* that may herald compression fractures

Note: Osteomalacia can produce the same symptoms as osteoporosis.

Traumatic Fractures of the Spine

- *Pain and local tenderness* may be the only features of undisplaced fracture.
- Palpable *gap* between spinous processes in the setting of trauma suggests unstable fracture.

Lumbar Spinal Stenosis

- Characteristic complaint is of *heaviness* or *numbness* of legs after modest exercise.
- Muscle weakness or decreased muscle stretch reflexes may be present immediately after exercise and normalize after rest.
- *Stoop test* is usually positive.

13

Male Genitalia and Rectum

Because gravity facilitates examination of the scrotum and examination for hernia, groin inspection and palpation are best done with patient upright and with you seated facing him. *Always wear gloves on both hands.* The inguinal area and genitalia must be fully exposed. Prostatic examinations proceed best with the patient bending over the end of the examination table (Fig. 13.1).

Genital examination is anxiety-provoking for many men. Be alert to the possibility of involuntary penile erection in response to genital manipulation, and if observed, address it directly and nonjudgmentally.

EXTERNAL GENITAL EXAMINATION

Goal. Determine abnormalities, if any, of the scrotum and phallus.

Technique. Inspect the skin of both the dorsal and ventral aspects of the penile shaft and prepuce for any lesions. In the uncircumcised, retract the foreskin to inspect all surfaces of the glans, noting its hygiene. Note the location of the urethral meatus. *Gentle* ventral-dorsal pressure applied to the glans promotes slight gaping of the urethral meatus to inspect its most anterior 1–2 mm for erythema or discharge.

Gently sliding the finger on the underside of the shaft and glans from the root of the penis to the tip may demonstrate urethral tenderness and can "milk" exudate not leaked spontaneously. After evaluation of the glans, corona, and urethral meatus, replace the foreskin.

Note the contour of each half of the scrotal sac. Elevate each hemiscrotum to inspect all surfaces for nodules, ulcerations, or discoloration.

Interpretation. Penile skin is usually darker than that elsewhere, so do not seek an abnormal pituitary-adrenal

265

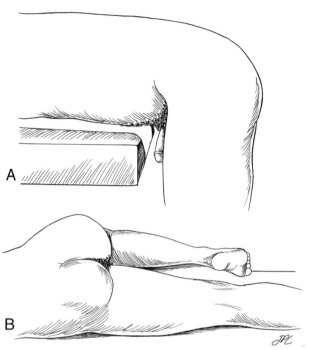

Figure 13.1 Positioning the patient for anorectal and prostate examination. **A.** For the patient who is able to bend over the examining table, this position works well. The perianal structures may be easily inspected by separating the buttocks (or asking the patient to use his hands to do this), and the rectum and prostate are readily palpated. **B.** For the patient who is less mobile, the left lateral decubitus position can facilitate anorectal and prostatic examination. Elevate the patient's right buttock with your left hand to expose the anal area. Insert the palpating finger of your right hand, with its palmar surface toward the ventral prostate gland, into the patient's anal orifice.

axis on the basis of darkening. The skin of the scrotal sac is also usually more deeply pigmented than elsewhere, thick, and heavily rugated.

Poor hygiene, particularly in uncircumcised men, predisposes to **balanoposthitis**, inflammation of the glans penis and overlying foreskin. Cases due to *Candida* tend to be the most intensely erythematous; balanoposthitis in which the scrotum is also involved or that includes small satellite nodules or papulopustules also suggests *Candida*. *Dermatophytes* may cause browner lesions, sometimes with central clearing. Persistent penile erythema after appropriate therapy for balanoposthitis raises the question of **squamous carcinoma in situ** (**erythroplasia** of Queyrat). An ulcerated, exophytic mass that appears stuck onto the penis or that replaces it is *invasive squamous cell carcinoma*.

Psoriasis commonly affects the penis, as does *Reiter's syndrome*, which can cause a noninfectious urethritis and striking inflammation of the glans, corona, and sulcus called *circinate balanitis*. A line of minute papules or fronds in parallel array around the coronal sulcus is indicative of the harmless *pearly penile papules*.

The classic nontender, painless solitary **penile ulcer** is the *chancre* of **syphilis**. In **gonorrhea**, physical findings may be absent or limited to an erythematous urethral meatus or diffuse urethral tenderness or expressible purulent discharge. Associated epididymal tenderness suggests that the same pathogen has ascended to the epididymis.

A red anterior urethra can occur in *anterior urethritis* from any cause, including excessive sexual intercourse. Sexual trauma can also reflect use of undue force during intromission, poor lubrication, or an inadequately distensible orifice. Its most extreme forms occur in cocaine users and include diffuse penile erythema, bite marks from incautious fellatio, ecchymoses, and hard, thrombosed, tender superficial penile veins. Overenthusiastic users of penile rings—legitimately prescribed for impotence—may also suffer penile injury.

Genital herpes simplex infection produces pain or paresthesia before the multiple minute vesicles on erythematous bases. Any part of the penis may be affected. In recurrent genital herpes, the lesions sometimes recur at the same spots. *Condylomata acuminata* result from infection with human **papillomavirus**. These **genital warts** favor the moistest areas, e.g., the corona and sulcus, although they may occur anywhere. They range from under 1 mm to about 1 cm across.

A foreskin that cannot be retracted constitutes **phimosis**. A retracted foreskin that cannot be brought forward to re-cover the glans is a **paraphimosis**.

An *apparently bent penis* usually indicates Peyronie's disease, a fibromatosis of the corpus cavernosum.

Hypospadias, a urethral orifice on the ventral surface of the glans or the penile shaft, can be innocent or can be associated with reduced fertility.

On palpation, the shaft of the normal penis feels uniformly flaccid and rubbery and is nontender.

The left hemiscrotum is often slightly longer than the right, giving an appearance of asymmetry. The scrotum and penis can swell if the iliac veins or lymph nodes are obstructed by tumor in the pelvis; in this case there will also be severe leg and thigh swelling. With *tense ascites*, intraperitoneal ascitic fluid can spread to cause prominent scrotal and/or penile swelling, so when this combination is present, a separate cause need not be sought. Common scrotal skin findings include minute bright-to-dark-red smooth-domed cutaneous hemangiomas, innocuous *Fordyce spots*. *Fournier's gangrene*, a life-threatening infection, produces extensive black necrosis of penile, scrotal, perineal, or perianal skin. Retroperitoneal hemorrhage can produce non-traumatic penoscrotal ecchymosis, *the blue genital sign of Bryant* in ruptured **abdominal aortic aneurysm**. With trauma, typically in a motor vehicle crash, a *butterfly-shaped hematoma* over the penis and scrotum is evidence of **urethral rupture**.

PALPATION OF SCROTAL CONTENTS

Goal. Assess the testes, epididymides, vasa deferentia, and other contents of the hemiscrota.

Technique. Palpate each side of the scrotal sac separately. Note any asymmetry in contents. Palpate each *testis* between your posteriorly placed palmar surfaces of the index through ring fingers and your anteriorly placed thenar eminence and thumb. From the upper to the lower pole, assess each hemiscrotal content for contour, masses, and areas of tenderness.

The head of the *epididymis* is usually located at the superoposterior pole of the testis. It is tubular, knobby, and separated from the body of the testis by connective tissue. As you examine each epididymis, compare it to the other regarding size, position, and tenderness. From the apex of the testis, the *vas deferens* courses cephalad into the inguinal canal. The vas is best found by gently bringing the palpating thumb and forefinger together at the top of the testis. The vas has the size and consistency of a pipe cleaner, although not its texture. The vas usually lies posteriorly, above the epididymis. Note the absence of a palpable vas, a rare but important sign. The other cord structures are not usually distinguishable from one another but make up a clump of soft strands accompanying the vas.

When the epididymis is hard to find, locate the vas as described, then move inferiorly until a more irregular structure than the smooth testis is encountered—this will be the epididymis.

If the scrotal contents are so retracted that palpation is impossible, give the patient time and warm the tissues; these measures reduce the involuntary muscle contraction that is responsible.

Interpretation. An *empty scrotum* signifies undescended or retracted testes, perhaps from nondescent and cryptorchidism. Smaller testes than normal are atrophic. Unilateral atrophy reflects remote injury. *Symmetric small firm testes* suggest Klinefelter's syndrome, cirrhosis-associated atrophy, HIV-associated testicular atrophy, remote trauma, orchitis, or pressure atrophy. Small soft testes suggest hypogonadotropic hypogonadism.

The normal adult testis is approximately 5 cm long and oval. The two testes should be of the same size; any appreciable size difference indicates abnormality. The consistency is moderately firm; palpation may elicit a visceral sensation experienced as diffuse pain. The surfaces of the testis are smooth, apart from the epididymis, and regular; any lump or other irregularity requires assessment. Testicular prostheses can feel very similar to the actual organ.

Orchitis, e.g., from mumps, produces a tender testis with or without enlargement.

If the vas cannot be found, the patient probably has agenesis or dysplasia of the vas, which carries a high association with ipsilateral renal agenesis. If normal vasa are felt, cystic fibrosis is excluded. After vasectomy, men often develop enlargement and firmness of one cut end, producing a nodule of *vasitis nodosum*.

A tender epididymis is characteristic of **acute epididymitis**. Sometimes, there is an associated urethritis. In the child with point tenderness over a spot on the testis or epididymis, consider **torsion of the appendix testis**.

An indurated nontender epididymis may represent tuberculosis.

SCROTAL MASSES AND TRANSILLUMINATION

Goal. Evaluate *(a)* any scrotal contents that are not expected structures or *(b)* abnormal portions of any such structures.

Technique.

1. In assessing an apparent testicular mass, the patient should be warm and comfortable, so that the testes hang freely to permit optimal palpation.
2. Try to feel a superior pole of the mass. If you can, you have excluded inguinal hernia, a mimic of testicular masses.
3. Auscultate the mass. Bowel sounds suggest hernia with small bowel in the hernia sac. If there are no sounds, no conclusion can be drawn.
4. *Transilluminate* the mass. This requires a dark room, with a strong, narrow light source held to the skin. Transilluminate the normal side first, to have a sense of the patient's baseline, and then repeat the test across the pathology. The light is held behind the hemiscrotum and directed forward. Observe from the front (Fig. 13.2): Cystic masses transmit light; solid masses do not.

Interpretation. Enlarged firm testes with minor tenderness, nontender enlarged testes, or testicular nodules sug-

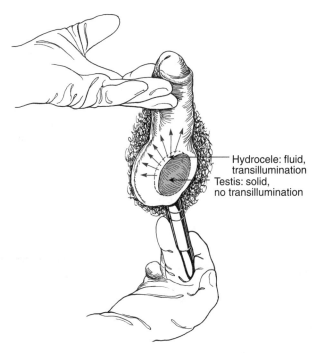

Figure 13.2 Transillumination of scrotal masses. With the room darkened, the penlight is held behind the mass and directed anteriorly. Failure to transmit light suggests solid tissue; transmission suggests a fluid-containing cyst.

gest **testicular neoplasm**. Soft, wormy, or yielding intrascrotal masses may represent various processes including hydrocele, varicocele, hernia, and epididymal cyst. But *do not dismiss testicular enlargement as inflammatory (non-neoplastic) because of tenderness*. In assessment of a testicular mass, the *absence of inguinal lymphadenopathy* offers *no* reassurance about nodal spread; the para-aortic lymph nodes are the usual site of metastases.

The epididymis usually lies on the posterolateral surface of each testis. In 7–10% of normal men, however, the epididymis lies anterior to the gland.

The most common scrotal enlargement is the *hydrocele*, a fluid accumulation in the cavity of the tunica vaginalis that forms a smooth, painless, resilient mass. It usually lies anterior to the testis. Transillumination verifies fluid content.

Varicocele's only adverse effect is reduced fertility. It feels like a "bag of worms." Because varicoceles are made up of blood-filled veins, they do *not* transmit light.

INGUINAL HERNIA EXAMINATION

Goal. Seek evidence of direct or indirect inguinal hernia and of femoral hernia. Besides patients seen for screening, any patient with **intestinal obstruction** needs a close search for entrapped hernias: direct inguinal, indirect inguinal, femoral, and ventral.

Technique. Observe the inguinal area for bulging or prominence. A cough, a laugh, or the Valsalva maneuver may bring out bulging. Palpation for inguinal hernia requires that you locate the pubic tubercles. Place the palmar surface of the index or middle finger directly over the area immediately lateral to each pubic tubercle, and ask the patient to cough or bear down. Feel for a single forceful pulsation against the finger, which suggests a defect in the fascia, permitting egress of a **direct inguinal hernia**.

Beginning well down at the most dependent point of one scrotal sac, gently insert the middle finger alongside the spermatic cord, invaginating the scrotal skin as the finger ascends the inguinal canal. With the palmar surface of the finger against the abdominal wall, the internal inguinal ring is felt as a depression above the inguinal ligament, 2–4 cm lateral to the pubic tubercle. Have the patient cough, with your finger in this position; a soft bulge descending along the canal suggests an **indirect inguinal hernia**.

To evaluate for **femoral hernia**, locate the femoral arterial pulse. With palmar surfaces of the index and middle fingers pressed into the femoral triangle just medial to the pulsation, have the patient cough. A soft bulge against your fingers suggests a femoral hernia.

Interpretation. Distinction of types is necessarily part of the description of technique, above. For anatomic discrimination between direct and indirect inguinal hernia presentations, see Figure 13.3.

ANORECTAL EXAMINATION

Goal. Assess the perianal skin and anorectal mucosa and wall for intrinsic anorectal abnormalities.

Technique. After completion of the genital and inguinal palpation, ask the patient to bend forward over the end of the examining table with legs slightly spread and elbows resting on the table (Fig. 13.1*A*). Optimal *visualization of perianal skin* calls for a modified Sims position. The patient extends the left hip and knee in contact with the examination table, flexes the right hip and knee, and finally turns the trunk and pelvis toward the table (Fig. 13.1*B*). With *both* hands gloved, retract the buttocks widely. This also optimizes illumination.

For tips on palpation, see Table 13.1.

To assess for **rectal prolapse**, have the patient bear down as though moving his bowels while buttock retraction is sustained.

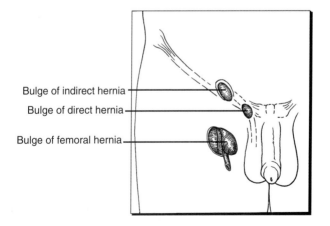

Bulge of indirect hernia
Bulge of direct hernia
Bulge of femoral hernia

Figure 13.3 Sites of presentation of indirect and direct inguinal hernias and of the infrequent male femoral hernia.

Table 13.1
Principles of Comfortable, Effective Rectal Examination

---

1. Do not stint on lubricant. Do not use water in place of a jelly for this purpose.
2. Reassure the patient. Have each action follow your words rather than accompanying or preceding them.
3. When you place your fingertip on the anal skin, leave it there unmoving for a moment. Then insinuate it gently and slowly.
4. Position the finger so that the sensitive *pad* is directed forward to the prostate to maximize the diagnostic accuracy of palpating this structure.

See Chapter 14 for more on examination of the anus and rectum.

Interpretation. Both gay and straight men can employ sexual anal penetration. In this setting, there may be perianal ecchymoses, lacerations, abrasions, loss of sphincter tone, *or, most typically, perfectly normal physical findings.* Many venereal lesions are found in the perianal skin. Chancres, herpetic vesicles, and condylomata resemble their penile counterparts. Progressive necrotizing **perianal herpetic infection** in HIV disease can cause large ragged ulcers and eschars.

Nontraumatic perianal ecchymosis has the same significance as its penoscrotal counterpart, i.e., retroperitoneal hemorrhage, as in the black-bottom sign after leakage from abdominal aortic aneurysm.

Perirectal abscesses are accompanied by severe pain and tenderness, erythema, or purulent drainage. They bulge, distorting perianal skin and contours, *without* prolapse having occurred.

Hemorrhoids in men resemble those in women. *External hemorrhoids* are smooth blue domes, often with surface erosions or ulcers, that are tender when inflamed or thrombosed. Their contour and surface are more regular than those of neoplasms. *Internal hemorrhoids*, above the anal verge, are rounded or elongated structures under a mucosa that feels intact. Pain from hemorrhoids is continuous, whereas pain on defecation is characteristic of **anal fissures**, minute shallow linear breaks in the epithelium, frequently without erythema, blood, or pus. Although tiny, they are exquisitely tender. **Perianal fistulas** are pathologic connections between the skin and the anal canal, usually from tissue destruction in neoplasia or Crohn's disease.

Rectal prolapse is extrusion of normal-appearing mucosa outside the anal verge. It commonly results from severe diarrhea and is accompanied by erythema, erosion, and maceration of perianal skin. Most rectal prolapses are readily *reducible* by simply pushing the tissue back in.

PROSTATIC EXAMINATION

Goal. Determine the presence and size of the prostate. Correlate features on palpation with any symptoms of urethral obstruction or of local inflammation. Discover any neoplasm of the prostate at its earliest, most curable stage.

Technique. Palpation of the prostate gland is performed with digital examination of the rectal vault, since the gland abuts the anterior part of the rectal ampulla. Its most proximal portion is reached by deep insertion of the gloved, lubricated middle finger. The prostate is characterized by bilobar shape and rubbery texture. After identifying the median raphe, which makes a central depression, palpate the rectal surfaces of each lobe, noting size, consistency, irregularities, or areas of tenderness. The lobes are normally symmetrical, and the rectal mucosa slides freely over them.

Try to determine, with any prostate nodule, whether induration extends beyond the gland and whether the prostate is mobile in the pelvis.

To reach higher on the prostate, use the middle finger, pressing the whole hand inward toward the navel while tightly flexing knuckles and interphalangeal joints of all fingers except the middle. This will compress the elastic subcutaneous fat and allow an extra centimeter of prostate to be reached; it will not hurt unless pressure is sudden or extreme.

Feel for *fluctuance* and localized prostatic tenderness. If prostatitis is under consideration, massage the prostatic fossa with the palpating finger several times.

After completion of the anorectal and prostatic examinations, provide the patient with tissue to wipe the perianal
area while you transfer stool on the withdrawn examining
finger to a card for inspection and occult-blood testing.

Interpretation. The prostate should be <4 cm across. The
lateral lobes should be symmetrical in size, shape, and consistency and be nontender. Diffuse enlargement of the
prostate, usually due to **benign prostatic hyperplasia**, is
common above age 60 and sometimes earlier. Prostatic
hyperplasia can occur without enlargement of the portion of
the gland accessible to palpation, so that *sometimes an anteri-
or median bar compromises urethral flow despite posterolateral
lobes that feel normal.* **Prostatic nodules** can occur in isolation
or with generalized prostatic enlargement. Many **prostatic
cancers** begin in the posterior lobe as hard nodules, but
other cancers arise out of reach or with a less distinctive texture. Several non-neoplastic conditions can also form nodules in the prostate (Table 13.2).

Table 13.2
Noncancerous Causes of Prostatic Nodules

Benign hyperplasia, often soft but sometimes hard
Calcinosis, especially with hard nodules
Prostatic infarct, complicating benign hyperplasia
Granulomatous prostatitis

Marked prostatic tenderness is a hallmark of **prostatitis**
and *prostatic abscess.* If pus drains from the urethra upon
prostatic palpation or massage, prostatitis is proven.

If a peritoneal shelf is palpable at the upper edge of the
prostate, suspect intraperitoneal carcinomatosis causing a
Blumer's shelf.

14

Female Genitalia and Rectum

The female rectal and the pelvic examination, with Papanicolaou smear, are an integral part of health maintenance of the normal adult female. In addition to this routine, there are specific indications for conducting the problem-focused pelvic and rectal examinations:

- Information obtained in the history, with or without symptoms
    1. Maternal diethylstilbestrol (DES) exposure
    2. Multiple (contemporaneous or serial) sexual partners
    3. Unexplained infertility
- New or recurrent sentinel symptoms
    1. Change in character, frequency, regularity, or dura tion of menses
    2. Midcycle, postcoital, or postmenopausal vaginal bleeding
    3. Lower abdominal pain or swelling, especially unilateral
    4. Painful sexual intercourse (dyspareunia)
    5. Vulvar or vaginal pruritus
    6. Change in quantity or character of vaginal discharge
    7. Urinary incontinence
    8. Burning or pain on urination (dysuria), with or without diagnosed urinary tract infection
    9. Lower back pain or any symptoms that bear consistent relationship to menstrual cycle
    10. Unexpected onset of menarche or menopause
    11. Bilateral lower limb edema (unexplained)
- New or recurrent rectal symptoms
    1. Blood in or on stool or on toilet paper or bleeding following defecation
    2. Pain in anorectum, either constant or on defecation
    3. New constipation or change in configuration of stool

      4. Perianal itching

      5. Melena

- Abnormalities detected on screening examination
  1. Skin lesions, swelling, or erythema of external genitalia
  2. Erythema, irritation, or mass of vaginal wall
  3. Erosion, friability, or mass on the cervix
  4. Enlargement, tenderness, immobility, or mass in uterus, ovary, salpinx, parametrium, or rectovaginal septum
  5. Perianal skin lesions or bleeding, tenderness, or mass in anus or rectum

Goal. Perform routine or symptom-specific pelvic evaluation.

Technique.

- Preparation
  1. Before positioning the patient, explain steps of the examination and answer questions.
  2. Have the patient empty her bladder.
  3. Have all supplies and equipment near at hand (Table 14.1).
  4. Determine that privacy is ensured.

Table 14.1
Instruments and Supplies

Examining table with	For Papanicolaou smears
Retractable stirrups	Bifid spatula
Padding for stirrups	Cotton swabs or endocervical brushes
Retractable foot tray	Glass slides/pencil
Flexible light source	Spray fixative
Examiner's stool or chair	For cervical/vaginal cultures and
Cloth drapes (sheets)	other studies for infection
Running warm water	Glass slides
Examination gloves,	KOH solution
disposable (nonsterile)	Saline solution
Assortment of speculum sizes	Thayer-Martin medium (for gonococci)
Hand mirror (for patient	Chlamydia transport medium
education)	Culturette tubes
Water-based lubricant	For fecal occult blood testing
	Smear cards (guaiac-impregnated)
	Developing fluid

5. Elevate the head of the table to 45°; pad the stirrups.
6. Adjust stirrup length to maximize patient comfort.
7. Ask the patient to push her buttocks toward the end of the table until she meets both your gloved hands positioned at the table edge.
8. Ask her to externally rotate her hips as far as is comfortable.
9. Drape as needed for warmth and comfort (see Fig. 14.1).
10. Sit down facing the patient's perineum.
- External genitalia (see Fig. 14.2)
    1. Inspect the external structures from anterior to posterior, using gentle retraction of labia to expose the underlying structures; ask the patient to bear down gently while you observe for bulging of anterior or

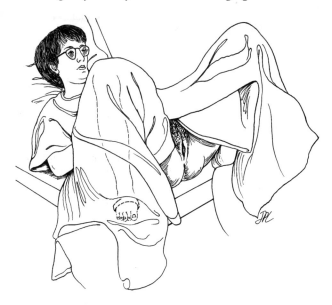

Figure 14.1 Patient positioned and draped for pelvic examination. Head of examining table is elevated 45° to permit eye contact between seated examiner and the patient. The drape covers the patient's thighs and legs.

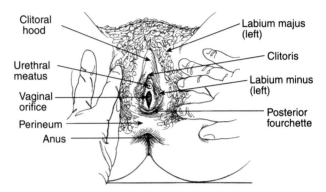

Figure 14.2 External female genitalia. In this view the urethral meatus, lying between the clitoris and the anterior part of the vaginal orifice (anterior fourchette), is mostly hidden in a labial fold. Note normal variant of redundant tissue of the right labium minus.

posterior vaginal walls into view and for drops of stress urinary leakage.

2. Retract the clitoral hood to inspect the clitoris for skin lesions.
3. Spread the labia minora to assess the urethral orifice for erythema or discharge.
4. Examine the vaginal orifice for patency.
5. Inspect the perineum for skin lesions or irritation.
6. Inspect the anal orifice for color, integrity, skin lesions, and venous prominences.
7. Palpate for enlargement of Bartholin's glands in the labia majora.
8. Palpate for enlargement of Skene's glands in the periurethral area.

• Vagina and cervix (inspection)
1. Moisten the appropriate-sized vaginal speculum with warm water.
2. With one finger in the posterior introitus, exert gentle downward traction (Fig. 14.3).
3. Introduce the closed speculum at 45° to the vertical.

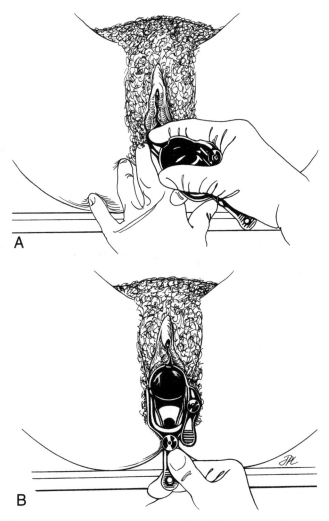

Figure 14.3 **A.** Insertion of vaginal speculum. The tip of the left index finger is inserted slightly into the posterior vaginal fourchette while exerting gentle downward traction. The right index finger rests on the superior blade of the speculum angled at 45° to the horizontal. **B.** After insertion of speculum blade tips, the instrument is rotated to the horizontal plane before opening of blades.

4. Direct the speculum toward the rectum as you pass it slowly into the vagina (Fig. 14.4).
5. When the full length of the blades has entered the vagina, rotate the speculum so its blades are at right angles to the introitus with the handle posterior.
6. Open the blades, watching for the cervix to "pop" into view between the tips of the blades.
7. Manipulate the blades until the cervical os is in full central view.
8. Fix the blades in full open position with the thumb screw.
9. Inspect the cervix for color, shape, friability, or bleeding.
10. Obtain desired cervical and vaginal samples (see below and Table 14.2).
11. Release the thumbscrew, slowly withdraw the speculum while rotating it to inspect vaginal mucosa for lesions, inflammation, or adherent discharge.

Table 14.2
Vaginal and Cervical Specimens for Smear and Culture

Purulent cervical discharge in sexually active patient
Consider: *Neisseria gonorrhoeae*
Procedure: With cotton swab, obtain cervical and vaginal secretions. For culture, spead specimen in "Z" pattern on Thayer-Martin plate or insert swab into culture tube.
Follow local instructions for labeling, transport, storage.
Cheesy white discharge with vulvar pruritus
Consider: *Candida albicans* (monilia) infection
Procedure: Obtain generous sample of discharge with swab, smear broadly on glass slide, mix with a drop of potassium hydroxide, add coverslip, examine immediately under microscope after brief gentle warming.
Watery, foul-smelling, copious discharge
Consider: *Trichomonas vaginalis* or *Gardnerella vaginalis*
Procedure: For trichomoniasis, collect vaginal pool specimen on spatula and transfer to glass slide; add 2 drops of saline solution, cover with glass coverslip, and examine promptly under microscope. For *G. vaginalis,* apply smear to dry slide and examine immediately under microscope.
Cervical erosion with surface purulence, urethritis with discharge, or history of exposure to infected male
Consider: *Chlamydia trachomatis*
Procedure: Several methods are currently available. Consult local laboratory.

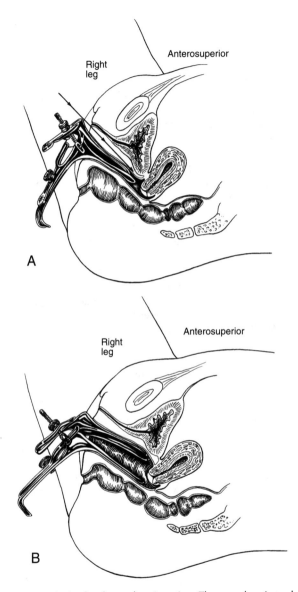

Figure 14.4 **A.** Angle of speculum insertion. The speculum is angled toward the sacrum as it is advanced along the vaginal canal toward the cervix. **B.** Once the speculum is inserted to its full length, the blades are slowly opened to expose the cervix to view and locked.

283

12. After the speculum has completely left the cervix, slowly close the blades during remaining witdrawal.
13. **Place the reusable speculum in a container designated for cleaning; place the disposable speculum directly into a disposal container.**

- Bimanual palpation of internal organs
    1. Remove glove from nondominant hand to be used for abdominal palpation.
    2. Stand between the stirrups facing the patient's perineum.
    3. Introduce the index and middle fingers of the gloved hand, palmar surfaces upward, into the introitus and pass them along the vaginal wall to the posterior fornix (see Fig. 14.5A).
    4. With the fingertips, palpate each fornix for tenderness, irregularities.
    5. Grasp the cervix between the fingertips and move laterally, seeking tenderness or fixation.
    6. With the fingers in the posterior fornix, elevate the cervix anteriorly.
    7. With the abdominal hand, feel for the elevated uterine fundus just above the symphysis pubis.
    8. With the fundus thus captured between your two hands, assess the uterus for size, smoothness of contour, mobility, tenderness.
    9. Place the internal fingers in one lateral fornix, projected parallel to the inguinal ligament toward the anterior superior iliac spine (Fig. 14.5B).
    10. Pressing downward, draw the abdominal hand slowly from the anterior superior iliac spine toward the symphysis, attempting to trap the ovary between your two hands.
    11. Repeat the motion, if necessary, to trap the elusive ovary; assess the ovary for size, tenderness, mobility, consistency.
    12. Examine the opposite adnexum in the same fashion.
- Anal and rectovaginal examination (Fig. 14.6)
    1. **Don fresh gloves** and sit again to directly visualize the anus.

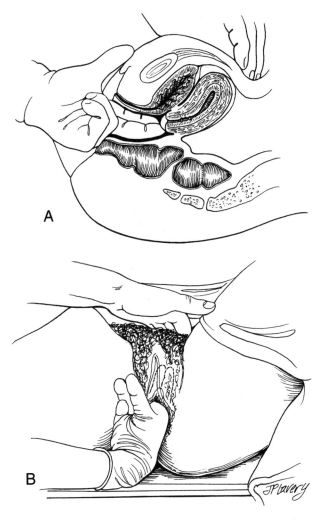

Figure 14.5 **A.** Uterine palpation. The two vaginal fingers find and elevate the cervix anteriorly, while the abdominal hand palpates the uterine fundus as it is pushed up from behind the pubic bone. **B.** Adnexal palpation. The intravaginal fingers press superolaterally into each adnexal region, while the abdominal fingers sweep parallel to the corresponding inguinal ligament, attempting to trap the ovary between the fingers of the two hands.

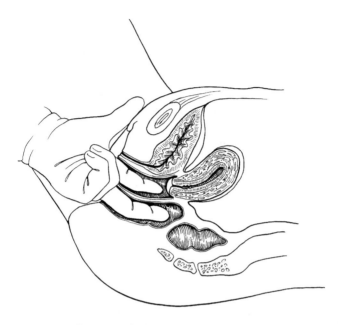

Figure 14.6 Rectovaginal examination. The rectovaginal septum is palpable between the two fingers as shown. The posterior surface of the uterus and cervix is palpated through the thin rectal wall. The fundus of a retroflexed uterus may be palpable only via the rectum.

2. Inspect the skin around the anus; with a finger on either side of the anus, spread the tissue laterally to visualize the surface of the anal pucker for bleeding, lesions, or cracks.
3. Lubricate the middle finger generously, place this tip at the anal verge, and ask the patient to bear down while you gently insert the finger into the anus.
4. Stand.
5. Introduce the index finger into the posterior aspect of the vagina such that the two internal fingers feel each other across the thin rectovaginal septum.
6. Sweep the approximated fingers side to side, feeling for tenderness or mass in the septum.

7. Remove the vaginal finger, keeping the rectal finger in place.
8. Palpate the posterior fundus of the uterus through the rectal wall. Assess for smoothness, mass, tenderness.
9. Palpate the rectum through a 360° sweep of the finger, feeling for mass or tenderness.
10. Remove the rectal finger and smear stool on the card for occult blood testing.
11. Help the patient to a sitting position, leave her with tissue and time to cleanse herself.

Interpretation.
- External genitalia
  1. Vulva

     Ulcers: venereal infection, granulomatous disease, neoplasm, drug eruptions, and vasculitis, e.g.,

     Behçet's syndrome

     Nevi: consider melanoma

     Generalized erythema: most commonly candidal vulvitis

     Masses: retention cysts (usually at the posterior introitus); condylomata acuminata (fleshy, frond-like papules caused by human papillomavirus); Bartholin's gland cyst and/or abscess (unilateral swelling in one labium majus)

  2. Urethral meatus

     Redness and swelling: local trauma (often sexual), urethral infection, or urethral caruncle; culture of discharge and careful history should help narrow possibilities

  3. Vaginal orifice (introitus)

     Prolapse of vaginal tissue through introitus: post-traumatic, as from childbirth, and loss of support; may be associated with cystocele and/or rectocele; these bulges appear at the anterior and posterior introitus, respectively, with Valsalva maneuver

Thinning with atrophy, punctate bleeding, or petechiae: estrogen deficiency; may progress to scarring and contraction of orifice

Erythema: candidal vaginitis

4. Anus and perianal skin:

Hemorrhoids: see Chapter 13, Male Genitalia and Rectum

Fissures: see Chapter 13, Male Genitalia and Rectum

Fistulae: fecal drainage and/or pus onto perianal skin

- Vagina and cervix (inspection)
  1. Uterine cervix

Normal mucosa pink; bluish in pregnancy

Small retention cysts on surface (Nabothian follicles): normal

Friable, ulcerated, eroded, or irregularly colored mucosa: sample for Papanicolaou smears and culture for *Chlamydia trachomatis*

Irregular, exophytic mass with necrotic surface: advanced cervical cancer

If you have any doubt about appearance of cervix, even with normal Papanicolaou smear and culture, refer for colposcopy and biopsy

Nulliparous os: a small pore near center of cervix

Parous os: slit-like or irregular

Red, pebbly-appearing endocervical tissue at rim of os: eversion

Soft, pink, smooth-surfaced mass at os: endocervical polyp

2. Vagina

Normal: pink, heavily rugated, and moist in reproductive age

Atrophy with diffuse friability: estrogen deficiency effects

Ulcers: same as for vulva (see Interpretation, 1. Vulva, above)

Inflammation: local trauma, irritation from use of external products such as deodorants or douches, from infection, e.g., candidal, trichomonal, or *Gardnerella* (see Table 14.2)

Localized mucosal abnormalities or masses: consider neoplasia

- Bimanual palpation of internal organs
  1. Uterus

     Cervix: may be deviated in any direction as variant uterine position; should be freely mobile without pain; consistency same as tip of nose but softens during pregnancy

     Uterine prolapse along vaginal canal:

       Grade 1: minor prolapse, apparent only with increased intra-abdominal pressure

       Grade 2: moderate prolapse, contained within vaginal canal but palpable without increased intraabdominal pressure

       Grades 3-4: prolapse external to introitus

     Normal variations in uterine position: see Figure 14.7

     Tenderness on manipulation: inflammation from infection or endometriosis

     Fixation to surrounding tissue: scarring from prior surgery or adnexal infection; suspicious for cancer, demands investigation/referral

     Enlargement: pregnancy, leiomyoma, or other neoplasia

     Serosal surface masses: leiomyomas (fibroid tumors)

  2. Adnexal structures

     Fallopian tubes: rarely palpable when normal; if one or both enlarged and tender consider infection; if one enlarged and tender, consider extrauterine pregnancy

     Ovaries: during reproductive years, 3 x 2 x 1 soft ovoids; decrease in size at menopause and then become nonpalpable; **a palpable ovary in a woman who is more than 3 years postmenopause is presumed neoplastic until proven otherwise**

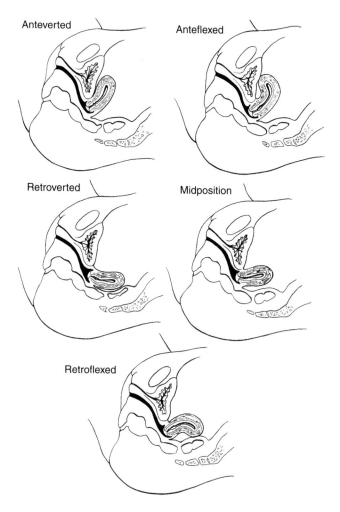

Figure 14.7 Range of normal uterine positions.

During childbearing years, enlargement suggests
benign cyst, polycystic ovary disease, or neoplasia

Unilateral enlargement is reassessed immediately after the next menses and examined by ultrasound if it has not diminished in size

- Anus and rectovaginal septum
  1. Anus

     Skin tags: suggest prior surgery or irritation

     Mass at anal verge: internal hemorrhoid, hypertrophied anal papilla, tumor

     Lax sphincter tone: childbirth trauma, selected neurologic disorders, local trauma, non specific during critical illness

     Mass or area of thickening and rigidity in anorectal area: cancer until proven otherwise
  2. Rectovaginal septum

     Normally a thin membrane, mobile and soft

     Rigidity or lumpiness: consider scar tissue, endometriosis, or carcinoma

OBTAINING CYTOLOGIC SAMPLES (PAPANICOLAOU)

1. Cervix and os are exposed to clear view through the speculum, which is locked open.
2. Insert a cytobrush or saline-soaked swab into the endocervix and twirl 360° to obtain *endocervical cells* (Fig. 14.8).
3. Immediately transfer the material to a clean, labeled glass slide; fix with spray or brief immersion in alcohol.
4. Insert the elongated end of the bifid cervical spatula into the os and scrape the surface of the cervix by rotating the spatula to obtain *exocervical cells*.
5. Immediately transfer material to a second clean and labeled glass slide and fix with spray as above.
6. Some clinicians also sample the *vaginal pool* for shed cells by dipping a swab into the posterior fornix and transferring material for processing as in step 3 above.

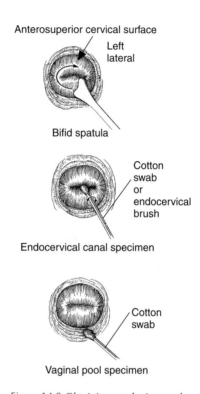

Figure 14.8 Obtaining cytologic samples.

PELVIC EXAMINATION IN SUSPECTED PREGNANCY

After the fourth to sixth week of gestation, any or all of the following signs may develop:

1. Bluish discoloration of the cervix (Chadwick's sign)
2. Soft generalized uterine enlargement
3. Focal uterine softening (Dickinson's sign)
4. Uterine pulsation

Note: Pelvic examination after the 24th week of gestation is conducted with great caution and *only* if indicated by abdominal or pelvic symptoms or under the supervision of an obstetrician.

EXAMINATION OF THE RAPE VICTIM

Although necessarily incomplete, the following principles apply:

1. Rape is a crime of violence, thus this examination must be conducted with the utmost gentleness and emotional support.
2. The purpose is twofold: to diagnose and treat any injury or infection; and to obtain evidence to convict a criminal.
3. Seek evidence of trauma in the genital area, mouth, anus, face, trunk, and limbs; take photograph (with patient's permission) if indicated.
4. Collect semen, even when dried (yellow-white and flaky), for use as evidence.
5. Do not assume the history is complete; presume that any part of the victim's body could have been violated.
6. Once diagnostic and legal data collections are complete, arrange for follow-up and for immediate interview and care by an experienced counselor.

Figure and Table Credits

Figure	Source
11.1	Reproduced with permission from Marshall Folstein, M.D.

Table	Source
2.12	Adapted with permission form American Heart Association. Recommendations for human blood pressure determination by sphygmomanometers. Dallas, Texas: American Heart Association, 1988. Copyright American Heart Association.
2.13	Adapted with permission from American Heart Association. Recommendations for human blood pressure determination by sphygmomanometers. Dallas, Texas: American Heart Association, 1988. Copyright American Heart Association.
10.4	Adapted form Sapira JP. The art and science of bedside diagnosis. Baltimore, Urban & Schwarzenberg, 1990.
10.13	Adapted form Sapira JP. The art and science of bedside diagnosis. Baltimore, Urban & Schwarzenberg, 1990.

Index

Page numbers in *italics* denote figures; those followed by "t" denote tables.

Abdomen, 169–192
  ascites evaluation, 186
  auscultation of, 172
  distension of, 182, 184–185
  inspection of, 171–172
  light palpation of, 173
  liver evaluation, 186–188, *187*
  masses of, 188–191, 190t
  normal consistency of, 176
  percussion of, 172
  quadrants of, 169, *170*
  regular palpation of, 173–177, 176t
  splenomegaly evaluation, 188
  surface landmarks of, 169
  surgical scars on, 171, *171*
  vascular abnormalities of, 192
  viscera of, 169–171
Abdominal pain, 173, 177–184
  causes of, 183t–184t
  examination for, 177–182
  guarding and rigidity, 179
  history taking for, 177
  interpretation of, 182–184
  rebound tenderness, 179
  visceral pain projections, 177, *178*
Abdominal reflexes, 248–249
Abdominojugular test
  for murmurs, 161–162
  for veins, 167
Abdominothoracic dyssynchrony, 128
Abducens nerve (CN VI), 81t, 88–90
Abscess
  Bartholin's gland, 287

  of breast, 123
  perirectal, 274
  prostatic, 276
Abstraction ability, 228
Abuse, examination of patients suffering physical or sexual, 21–22
Accessory nerve (CN XI), 81t, 113, *113*
Achilles reflex, 246–247, *247*, 261
Achilles tendon, 223
Acne, 56t
Acoustic nerve (CN VIII), 81t, 93–96
Acrocyanosis, 196–197
Adie's syndrome, 87
Adrenocortical insufficiency, 142
Advance directives, 31
Affect, 227
Age
  looking older than, 34t
  looking younger than, 33t
Agnosia, 230
Agraphia, 230
Aird's test, 262
Alcohol use history, 6
  extended, 20–21
Allen's test, 195–196, *196*
Allergic rhinitis, 76–77
Allergies, 5
Alopecia, 59t
Amyl nitrite test, 161
Angular cheilosis, 79
Anisocoria, 69, 87
Ankle, 221–223
  arthritis of, 222

Ankle–*continued*
   Charcot's, 221, 221t
   dependent edema of, 222
   mortise, 223
   muscle and nerve control of
      motion of, 217t
   reduced power of, 221
   testing range of motion of, 221
Ankylosing spondylitis, 263
Anomia, 230
Anorectal examination, 180, 274t
   female, 284–287, *286*, 290–291
   male, *266*, 273–275
Anorexia nervosa, 80
Anorgasmia, 18–19
Antalgic gait, 219
Anterior cruciate ligament,
   219–220
Aorta, 170
   aneurysms of, 183t, 192, 268
   palpation on sides of, 174
Aortic insufficiency, 155–156,
   159–160
Aortic stenosis, 142, 143, 148,
   150, 155–156
Aphasia, 230, 232
Aphthous stomatitis, 79
Apical cardiac impulse, 141–143
Apley scratch test, 201t
Appearance, 33, 33t–34t
Appendicitis, 183t–184t
Apraxia, 231, 232
Arcus cornealis, 69
Arm. *See* Upper limb
Arrhythmia, sinus, 146
Arthritis
   ankle, 222
   hand, 206–207
   metatarsophalangeal, 223, 224
Asbestosis, 26
Ascites, 172, 186, 268
Asterixis, 209–210, 243

Ataxia, 250
Athetosis, 243
Athlete's foot, 65t
Atonia, 242
Atrial fibrillation, 167
Atrial septal defect, 149
Atrophy
   muscle, 242
   skin, 52
   testicular, 269
   vaginal, 20, 288
Auscultation, 10
Autonomic dysfunction, 44t
Axilla. *See* Breasts and axillae

Babinski response, 249
Back, lower, 251–264
   causes of pain of, 262–264
      ankylosing spondylitis,
         263
      herniated intervertebral
         disc or disc fragments, 262
      lumbar spinal stenosis,
         264
      lumbosacral strain, 263
      osteoarthrosis, 263
      osteoporosis, 263
      spinal fractures, 264
      spondylolisthesis, 263
   evaluating pain of, 255–262
      due to neurologic
         abnormalities, 260t
      examination with patient
         prone, 261
      examination with patient
         sitting, 261
      examination with patient
         supine, 259–261
      extended maneuvers for,
         258t
      palpation with patient
         standing, 258

Schober's flexion test, 256, *259*

stoop test for entrapment radiculopathy, 261

tests for malingering, 262

hip extension, 254, *257*

inspection and palpation of, 251–252, *252*

normal alignment of, 251–252, *252*

spinal curvatures, 252–254, *253*

spinal range of motion, 254, *255–256*

surface landmarks of, *252*

Balanoposthitis, 266–267

Ballottement, 220t

Barrel chest, 126

Bartholin's glands, 280

Basal cell cancer, 62t

Bedsores, 64t

Bench test, 262

Benign prostatic hyperplasia, 276

Biceps reflex, 246

"Birthmarks," 55t

Black bottom sign, 274

Bladder, urinary, 171, 177

distension of, 189

Blisters, 57t

Blood pressure measurement, 37–45

bilateral upper limb, 194

causes of artifacts in, 41t

contraindications to using limb for, 43t

discrepant side-to-side readings from, 40

interpretation of, 40

orthostatic pulse and, 41–45

caveats for, 44–45

contraindications to, 42

deconditioning and, 43

interpretation of, 43

orthostatic tachycardia, 43

technique for, 42–43

patient characteristics affecting, 42t–43t

problems and solutions for, 40–41

sources of variation in, 42t

technique for, 38–40

Blue genital sign of Bryant, 268

Blumer's shelf, 276

Bouchard's nodes, 207

Bowel obstruction, 182

Bowel palpation, 176

Bowlegs, 219

Brachioradial delay, 195

Brachioradialis reflex, 246

Bradycardia, sinus, 35t, 145

Bradykinesia, 244

Breasts and axillae, 115–124

abscess, 123

axillary lymphadenopathy, 117–118, 123–124

breast cancer, 63t, 122–124

male, 123

breast texture, 121–122

cysts, 122

effect of movement on, 116

fibrocystic breasts, 121

history taking related to, 115

inspection of, 115–118

male, 119, 123

masses of, 119–120, 122–123

nipples, 118, 121

Paget's disease, 63t, 121

palpation of, 118–119, *119*

positions to observe for asymmetry of, *117*

during pregnancy and lactation, 120–122

skin abnormalities of, 63t

Breasts and axillae—*continued*
supernumerary breasts, 120
Tanner stages of breast
development, *116*
timing for examination of, 115
unilateral breast enlargement,
121
venous pattern of breasts, 120
visible attributes of, 120
Breath sounds. *See also* Lung;
Respiration
abnormal, 135–136
normal, 135t
Broca's aphasia, 230
"Brownout," 44
Brown-Sequard syndrome, 239t
Brudzinski's contralateral
reflex signs, 234t
Brudzinski's nape of neck sign,
234t
Bruises, 50
Bruits
abdominal, 192
carotid artery, 105, 164
subclavian artery, 104
vertebral artery, 104
Buccal mucosa, 78–80
Buerger's test, 211–212
Bulge test, 220t
Bulimia, 80
Bullae, 52, 57t
Bullous myringitis, 75
Bullous pemphigoid, 57t
Bundle branch block, 149
Bunions, 224

Café-au-lait spots, 55t
Calluses, 56t
Caloric testing of comatose
patient, 95–96
Cancer, carcinoma
anorectal, 291

basal cell, 62t
breast, 63t, 122–124
cervical lymph nodes as
markers for, 109–110
liver, 187–188
oral, 79–80
ovarian, 289
prostate, 276
skin, 62t
squamous cell, 62t, 267
testicular, 271
thyroid, 106
Candida infections
oral, 79, 80
penile, 266–267
stomatitis, 79
vaginal, 287
vulvar, 287
Cardiac impulses, 141–143
Carpal tunnel syndrome, 209
Carrying angle, 203
Carvallo's sign, 160
Cat-scratch disease, 110, 117–118
Cauda equina syndrome, 235
Cellulitis, 65t, 68, 214, 215t
Central venous pressure, 165
Cerebellar disease, 244
Cerebellar testing, 249–250
Cerebral function. *See*
Neurologic examination
Cerumen removal, 76
Cervical lymph nodes, *107–109,*
107–110
enlarged, 109
fixed, 110
generalized lymphadenopathy,
110
hard, 109–110
massive, 110
soft, fluctuant, 110
Cervical masses, 110–112, *111*

Cervical spine, 20, 101–104
  cervical spinal root disease,
    103–104
  compression test of, 103
  movement abnormalities of,
    101–102
  normal gentle extension
    curve of, 101
  quadrant test of, 103
  range of motion of, 101, *102*
  tenderness to percussion, 102
Cervical venous hums,
  104–105, 164
Cervix, uterine, 280–284, *281,
  283*
  abnormalities of, 288
  palpation of, 284
Chaddock reflex, 249t
Chadwick's sign, 291
Chancre, 64t, 267
Charcot's joints, 221, 221t
Cheilosis, angular, 79
Chemosis, 69
Chest wall observation, 125–128
Chickenpox, 57t
Chief complaint (CC), 2
Child abuse, 22
Childhood illnesses, 5
Chlamydia trachomatis, 288
Chloasma, 55t
Cholecystitis, 183t, 184
Chorea, 243
Circinate balanitis, 267
"Clasp-knife" phenomenon, 242
Clavicle, unilateral prominent,
  202
Clawtoe, 224
Clicks, 150
Clitoris, 280
Clubbing, 58t
Cocaine use, 86, 267
Coen's test, 203, 204

Cogwheel rigidity, 208, 242, 244
Colonic obstruction, 182
Colostrum, 121
Coma, 233
Common cold, 77
Compression test, 103
Concentration ability, 227
Condylomata acuminata, 267,
  287
Conjunctiva
  abnormalities of, 69–70
  inspection of, 70
Conjunctivitis, 92
Corneal sensitivity, 91–92
Corns, 56t
Cortical disease, 231
Costochondritis, 129
Costovertebral angle palpation,
  129
Coxsackievirus, 60t
Crackles, 136
Cranial nerve (CN) evaluation,
  81t–82t, 81–98, 227,
  233–234
  abducens nerve (CN VI),
    88–90
  accessory nerve (CN XI), 113,
    113
  acoustic nerve (CN VIII),
    93–96
  facial nerve (CN VII), 92–93
  glossopharyngeal nerve (CN
    IX), 96–97
  hypoglossal nerve (CN XII),
    97–98
  mnemonic for, 81
  oculomotor nerve (CN III),
    84–88
  olfactory nerve (CN I), 82–83
  optic nerve (CN II), 83–84
  trigeminal nerve (CN V),
    90–92, *91*

Cranial nerve (CN) evaluation–
    continued
    trochlear nerve (CN IV),
        88–90
    vagus nerve (CN X), 96–97
Cremasteric reflex, 248–249
Crohn's disease, 80
Cruciate ligaments, 219–220
Crust, 52
Cryptorchidism, 269
Cullen's sign, 184
Cyanosis, 125, 196
Cycled respiration test, 160
Cystic hygroma, 111
Cysts, 52
    Bartholin's gland, 287
    branchial cleft, *111*
    breast, 122
    epidermal inclusion
        (sebaceous), 56t, 67, 204
    ganglion, 204
    ovarian, 186
    pilonidal, 64t
    retention, 287, 288
    thyroglossal duct, 111, *111*
Cytomegalovirus, 110

Dahl's sign, 125
de Quervain's chronic
    stenosing tenosynovitis, 207
Decarboxyhemoglobinemia,
    196
Depression, 24
Dermatitis
    eczematous contact, 57t
    herpetiformis, 57t
    inframammary, 63t
    seborrheic, 56t, 62t
    venosa, 65t, 213
Dermatoliposclerosis, 213
Dermatomes, 236, *237*
Dermatomyositis, 206

Diabetes
    Charcot joints in, 221
    foot ulcers in, 65t, 223, 224
    shin spots in, 65t
Diaphragm motion, 132–134
Diascopy, 48, 54
Diastasis recti, 173
Diastole, 150–152
Diastolic murmurs, 155
Dickinson's sign, 291
Diet and nutritional history, 6
    extended, 26–29
        based on abnormal
            laboratory tests, 28–29
        based on signs from
            physical examination,
            27–28
        for concerns raised by
            clues in other portions
            of screening history, 27
        indications for, 26–27
Digiti quinti sign, 239, 243
Diverticulitis, 184t
Diverticulum, 111
Dorsiflexion, 221, 259
Driving and drinking, 21
Drugs
    effect on pupil size, 86
    hypersensitivity reactions to,
        57t, 60t
    rashes induced by, 61t
"Dry skin," 55
Dupuytren's contracture, 206
Dysarthria, 228–230, 232
Dyspareunia, 18
Dysphonia, 230, 232
Dystonia, 243

Ears, 73–75, 73–76
    cerumen removal, 76
    external
        abnormalities of, 75

examination of, 73, *74*
external auditory canal, 75
otoscopic examination, 73–75
tympanic membrane, *74, 75*
Ecchymosis, 50
perianal, 274
Ectropion, 69
Eczema, 57t
Edema
ankle, 222
causes of, 214t
facial, 68–69
lower limb, 212t, 212–213
Egophony, 139
Ejection clicks, 150
Elbow, 203–204
carrying angle of, 203
Coen's test of, 203, 204
muscle and nerve control of
motion of, 201t
palpating for effusion at, 203
reduced power of, 203
subcutaneous nodules at,
203, 204
testing range of motion of,
203
Elder abuse, 22
Emphysema, subcutaneous, 129
Enanthems, 61t
Enteroviruses, 60t
Entrapment radiculopathy, 261
Environmental health history,
24–26
Ephelides, 62t
Epidermolysis bullosa, 57t
Epididymis, 269, 271
Epididymitis, 270
Epstein-Barr virus, 110
Erosions, 52, 56t
Erysipelas, 57t
Erythema
nodosum, 65t

pharyngeal, 80
Erythrasma, 65t
Erythromelalgia, 212
Erythromelia, 211
Erythroplasia of Queyrat, 267
Ethmoid sinus fracture, 68
Exanthems, 61t
Exfoliative erythroderma, 61t
Exophthalmos, 69–70
Extended examination, 13–31
Eye and periorbital structures,
69–73
conjunctival abnormalities,
69–70
eye movements, 88–90, *89*
apparent deficits of, 89–90
eyelid abnormalities, 69
funduscopic examination,
71–72
inspection of superior
conjunctiva, 70
"nipple" test, *70,* 70–71
normal variants, 69
pupillodilation, 72–73
visual acuity testing, 83
visual field defects, 84
visual field testing, 83

Face
examination of, 67–69
sensory perception to light
touch and pain, 90
Facial dysmorphism, 68
Facial nerve (CN VII), 81t, 92–93
Fallopian tubes, 289
Family (medical) history (FH), 7
Family violence history, 22–23
Fat embolism, 60t
Femoral artery, 175
Fever
causes of, 38t
in critical care unit, 39t

Fever–*continued*
  detection of, 36–37
  extreme pyrexia, 39t
  hemorrhagic rashes and
    lesions in patients with, 60t
  without tachycardia, 38t
Fibroadenoma of breast, 122
Fingers
  deformities of, 206t
  muscle and nerve control of
    motion of, 202t
  tests for, 209
Finkelstein's test, 207
Fissures
  anal, 64t, 274–275
  epidermal, 53
Fistulas, perianal, 64t, 275
Flaccidity, 242
Flatfoot, 223
Fluctuation test, 220t
Folstein Mini-Mental Status
  Examination, 228, 229, 232
Foot, 221–226
  diabetic ulcers on, 65t, 223,
    224
  skin abnormalities of, 65t
Forced expiratory time, 138
Fordyce spots, 64t, 268
Fournier's gangrene, 268
Fractures, spinal, 264
Fremitus, 136–138, 137
"Frigidity," 18
Frontal bossing, 67
Frontal lobe signs, 231t
Funduscopic examination, 71–72

Gait assessment, 219, 225,
  244–245, 245
Galactocele, 123
Gallavardin phenomenon, 156
Gallbladder, 169
  masses of, 191

Gallops, 151, 152
Gangrene, 65t
Gardner's syndrome, 67
General appearance, 33, 33t–34t
Genital examination, 182
  female, 277–293
    bimanual palpation of
      internal organs, 284,
      285, 289, 290
    external genitalia,
      279–280, 280, 287–288
    indications for problem-
      focused examination,
      277–278
    instruments and supplies
      for, 278t
    obtaining cytologic
      samples, 291, 292
    patient positioning for,
      278–279, 279
    preparation for, 278–279
    rape victim, 292–293
    suspected pregnancy,
      291–292
    vagina and cervix,
      280–284, 282t, 288
  male, 265–276
    external genitalia, 265–268
    inguinal hernia, 272–273,
      273
    patient positioning for,
      265, 266
    prostate, 275–276, 276t
    scrotal masses and
      transillumination,
      270–272, 271
    scrotal palpation, 268–270
Genital warts, 64t, 267
Genu recurvatum, 219
Genu valgum, 219
Genu varum, 219
Gingivae, 78–80

Gland(s)
    Bartholin's, 280
    Montgomery, 120
    prostate, 275–276
    Skene's, 280
    thyroid, 99, 105, 105–106
Glossitis, 79
Glossopharyngeal nerve (CN
    IX), 81t, 96–97
Glove-and-stocking
    neuropathy, 235
Gluteus medius strength
    testing, 216–217, 218
Gonorrhea, 60t, 80, 267
Gooch's test, 160
Gordon reflex, 249t
Gottron's sign, 206
Gout, 203, 204, 223, 224
Graham Steell murmur, 155
Graphesthesia, 230–231
Graves' disease, 69–70, 106, 110
Great artery assessment, 162–164
    carotid murmurs, 163–164
Great vein assessment, 165–168
    abdominojugular test for
        veins, 167
    Kussmaul's sign, 168
Grey Turner's sign, 184
Gynecomastia, 123

Hair alterations, 59t
Hairy leukoplakia, 79, 80
Half-and-half nails, 58t
Hallux
    extension of, 221
    valgus, 224
Hammertoe deformity, 224
Handgrip test, 158
Hands
    examination of, 205t–206t,
        205–207
    "flapping" of, 210

tests for, 209
    tremor in, 208, 208t
Head
    examination of, 67
    lymphatic drainage of, 108
    skin problems of, 62t
Health habits, 6
Hearing examination, 93–96,
    94t, 96t
Hearing Handicap Inventory
    for the Elderly, 93–95, 94t
Heart, 141–168
    auscultation of, 143–156
        adverse effects of
            examining through
            clothing, 145, 146t
        diastole, 150–152
        first heart sound, 146–148,
            147
        fourth heart sound, 151,
            151–152
        heart murmurs, 143,
            152–156, 153t
        interpretation of rate and
            rhythm, 145–146
        second heart sound, 147,
            148–149
        sites for, 143–145, 144
        systole, 150
        technique for, 143–145
        third heart sound, 151,
            151–152
    inspection of cardiovascular
        motion, 141
    manipulations of murmurs
        and heart sounds, 156–162
        abdominojugular maneuver
            for murmurs, 161–162
        amyl nitrite test, 161
        aortic insufficiency
            maneuvers, 159–160

Heart–*continued*
  body position maneuvers, 157
  cycled respiration test, 160
  handgrip test, 158
  locale and transmission, 156–157
  passive straight-leg raising maneuver, 159
  transient arterial occlusion maneuver, 160–161
  Valsalva maneuver, 157–158
  palpation of, 141–143
    apical impulse, 141–143
    technique for, 141–142
    thrills, 143
Heaves, 142
Heberden's nodes, 207
Heel-to-shin maneuver, 250
Heliotrope sign, 62t
Hemangioma, cherry, 56t
Hemianopsia, 84, 234
Hemiballism, 243
Hemiparesis, 225–226
Hemochromatosis arthropathy, 207
Hemorrhoids, 64t, 274
Hepatomegaly, 173, 187
Hernia, 179, *180*, 185
  femoral, 272, *273*
  inguinal, 272–273, *273*
Herniated disc, 262
Heroin, 86
Herpes simplex virus, 57t
  genital, 57t, 64t, 267
  intraoral, 79
  perianal, 274
Herpes zoster virus, 57t, 92
Hidradenitis suppurativa, 63t
Hip, 215–219
  extension of, 254, *257*

  flexion contracture of, 217–219
  muscle and nerve control of motion of, 217t
  reduced power of, 216
  testing range of motion of, 215–216
History of present illness (HPI), 2–4
HIV history, 29–31
  patient concerns, 29
  patient with known HIV infection, 30–31
  risk assessment, 29
  unexplained physical findings, 30
HIV infection, 30–31
  frontal bossing in, 67
  generalized lymphadenopathy in, 110
  oral manifestations of, 80
Holosystolic murmurs, 143, 155
Hoover's test, 225–226
Hordeolum, 69
Hospitalizations, 4–5
"Hot flashes," 55
Household toxin exposure, 26
Human papillomavirus, 267, 287
Hydrocele, 272
Hydrocephalus, 67
Hyperpnea, 126
Hypertension, 142, 148
Hyperventilation, 126
Hypervigilance, 233
Hypoglossal nerve (CN XII), 81t, 97–98
Hypospadias, 268
Hypotension, orthostatic, 43–44, 44t
Hypotonia, 242, 244
Hypovolemia, 43–45, 45t

Ileocecal obstruction, 182
Ileus, 182
Iliac crests, 169, 251
Iliac spine
    anterior superior, 169
    posterior superior, 251
Iliopsoas maneuver, 180, *181,* 184
Immunizations
    for HIV-infected persons, 31
    status of, 5–6
Impetigo, 57t
Impotence, 17
Incisions, abdominal, *171*
Inguinal ligament, 169, 174–175
Inspection, 10
Intervertebral disc herniation,
    262
Intestinal obstruction, 179, 182,
    183t, 272
Intracranial pressure, 233
Involuntary movements, 242–244
Iridodonesis, 69

Janeway lesions, 194
Jendrassik maneuver, 245, *246*
Joint position sense, 236–238
Jugular venous pressure,
    165–168

Kaposi's sarcoma, 62t, 80
Keloid, 56t
Keratosis
    seborrheic, 56t, 62t
    solar (actinic), 56t, 62t
Kernig's sign, 234t
Kidney, 170
    "capturing" of, 189–190
    enlarged, 189
    masses of, 191
    palpation of, 174, 177
Klinefelter's syndrome, 269
Klippel-Feil anomaly, 100

Knee, 219–220
    deformities of, 219
    detecting effusions of, 220t
    draw(er) tests for, 220
    muscle and nerve control of
        motion of, 217t
    reduced power of, 219
    testing range of motion of,
        219
Knock-knee, 219
Knuckle pads, 206
Knuckle sign, 207
Kocher incision, *171*
Korotkoff sounds, 40–41
Kussmaul's sign, 168
Kyphosis, 127, *253,* 254

Labia minora and majora, 280
Lactation, 120–121
Ladder sign, 182
Language, 228–231
Laryngocele, 112
Lasègue sign, 234t
Leg. *See* Lower limb
Leiomyomas, uterine, 289
Lens, 71
Lentigines, 55t, 62t
Lentigo maligna, 62t
Lethargy, 233
Leukemia, 110
Level of consciousness, 227, 233
Libido, loss of, 18
Lichenification, 56t
Limbs, 193–226
    examination principles for,
        193t, 193–194
    lower, 210–226
    upper, 194–210
Line(s)
    Beau's, 58t
    Mees', 58t
    "milk," 120

Lipomas, 56t, 67, 173
Lips, 77–79
Liver, 169
    enlarged, 173, 187
    hard, 187
    masses of, 191
    palpation of, 173, 174, *175*,
        176
    percussion of, 172
    scratch test to define lower
        border of, 186–187, *187*
    tumors of, 187–188
Lordosis, *253*, 254
Lower limb, 210–226
    arterial, venous, and capillary
        circulation of, 210–213, *211*
    edema of, 212t, 212–213, 214t
    joints, tendons, muscles, and
        bones of, 215–225
        ankle and foot, 221–222
        feet and toes, 222–225
        hip, 215–219
        knee, 219–220, 220t
    leg length discrepancy, 251–252
    lymphatic drainage of, 213–214
        muscle and nerve control
            of joint motion, 217t
    painful and swollen, 212, 213t
    paralysis of, 225–226
    peripheral nerves and
        muscles of, 225–226, 250
    skin abnormalities of, 65t
        Tinetti functional test, 215,
            216t
Lower motor neuron lesions,
    243, 243t
Lumbosacral strain, 263
Lung, 125–139
    auscultation of, 134–136
        abnormal breath sounds,
            135–136
        auscultatory percussion,
            138–139
        egophony, 139
        normal breath sounds, 135t
        pectoriloquy, 139
        posttussive/post-deep-
            breathing, 138
        technique for, 135
    forced expiratory time, 138
    hyperinflation of, 142
    percussion of, 130–134
        for diaphragmatic motion,
            132–134
        lung apex, 134
        percussion notes, 132, *133*
        posterior and lateral
            lungs, 131–132
        sites for, *131*
        technique for, *130*, 130–131
    positional signs of chronic
        disease of, 125
Lunulae, red, 58t
Lurching gait, 219
Lymph nodes
    cervical, *107–109*, 107–110
    epitrochlear, 197
    head and neck, *108*
    inguinofemoral, 174, 213–214
    popliteal, 213
    subhumeral, 197
Lymphadenopathy
    axillary, 117–118, 123–124
    cervical, 109–110
    epitrochlear, 197
    generalized, 110
    inguinal, 271
Lymphangitic streaking, 214
Lymphoma, 110

Macrognathia, 68
Macules, 49, 55t
Malar rash, 62t

Male pattern baldness, 59t
Malignant melanoma, 62t, 63t
Malingering, 262
Mandibular nerve (CN V3), *91*, 92
Mann's test, 220t
Masses
    breast, 119–120, 122–123
    intraabdominal, 188–191, 190t
    neck, 110–112, *111*
    scrotal, 270–272, *271*
    vulvar, 287
Masseter muscles, 90
Mastitis, 63t, 121
Maxillary nerve (CN V2), *91*, 92
McBurney incision, *171*
Measles, 60t
Median nerve damage, 209
Mediastinal crunches, 150
Medical history, 1–9
    chief complaint, 2
    components of, 3t
    definition of, 1
    extended, 14–31
        definition of, 14
        diet and nutritional history, 26–29
        environmental health history, 24–26
        family violence history, 22–23
        HIV history, 29–31
        mental health history, 23–24
        process for, 14, 15t
        settings calling for, 14
        sexual history, 15–20
        substance use history, 20–22
    facilitators of, 1
    family history, 7
    history of present illness, 2–4
    past medical history, 4–6
    patient profile, 6–7
    process guidelines for, 2t
    review of systems, 7–10
    screening, 1–9
Medications, 5
Memory testing, 228
Meningeal irritation, 233, 234t
Meningococcemia, 60t
Mental health history, 23–24
Metabolic encephalopathy, 209–210
Metacarpophalangeal joint inflammation, 205
Metatarsophalangeal arthritis, 223
Micrognathia, 68
Mitral prolapse, 150, 154–155, 157
Mitral regurgitation, 143, 151, 158, 161
Mitral stenosis, 147, 151, 152, 155
Molluscum contagiosum, 57t
Mononeuropathy, 235
Monoparesis, 225–226
Montgomery glands, 120
Mood, 227
Motor evaluation, 239, 242–245
    gait assessment, 244–245, *245*
    interpretation of, 243–244
    involuntary movements, 242–243
    technique for, 239, 242–243
Mouth. *See* Oral cavity
Murphy's sign, 180, 184
Muscle atrophy, 242
Muscle fasciculations, 236, 242
Muscle strength testing, 242, 242t
Muscle stretch reflexes, 235, 245–247, *246–247*, 248t

Muscle tone, 242
Muscle weakness, 235
  degree of, 242, 242t
  distribution of, 239
Myringitis, bullous, 75

Nabothian follicles, 288
Nail alterations, 58t
  of toenails, 223–225
Navel
  position of, 169
  protuberant, 171–172
Neck, 99–113
  anatomy of, *99*
  blood vessels of, 104–105
  cervical lymph nodes,
    107–109, 107–110
  cervical spine, 101–104
  general assessment of, 99–100
  masses in, 110–112, *111*
  "neck sign," 101
  short, webbed, 100
  skin problems of, 62t
  thyroid gland, *99, 105,* 105–106
  torticollis, 100
  trachea, 112
  triangles of, *100*
Neurologic examination,
  227–250
  cerebellar testing, 249–250
  cranial nerve evaluation,
    81–98, 233–234
  head and intracranial status,
    233
  integrative cerebral function,
    227–233
    abstraction, 228
    cerebral functional
      localizations, *232*
    Folstein Mini-Mental
      Status Examination,
      228, *229,* 232

frontal lobe signs, 231t
interpretation, 231–233
language and speech,
  228–231
level of consciousness, 233
memory, 228
reasoning, 228
motor evaluation, 239–245
  gait assessment, 244–245,
    245
  involuntary movements,
    242–243
  upper vs. lower motor
    neuron disease, 243, 243t
reflexes, 245–249
  muscle stretch reflexes,
    245–247, *246–247,* 248t
  superficial reflexes,
    248–249, 249t
sensory evaluation, 236–239
signs of meningeal irritation,
  233, 234t
spinal cord, nerve root, and
  peripheral nerve
  function, 234–236
supplies and equipment for,
  227t
Nevus, 55t
  melanocytic, 62t
  vulvar, 287
Nicotine stains on nails, 58t
"Nipple" test, *70,* 70–71
Nipples, 118, 121
  rudimentary, 120
Nodes
  Bouchard's, 207
  Heberden's, 207
  lymph. *See* Lymph nodes
  Osler, 207
Nodules, 51, 56t
  prostatic, 276, 276t
  rheumatoid, 203, 204

Nose, 68, 76–77
Nystagmus, 96, 208, 250

Obturator maneuver, 180, *181*, 184
Oculomotor nerve (CN III), 84–88
Ogilvie's syndrome, 182
Olecranon bursitis, 203
Olfactory nerve (CN I), 81t, 82–83
Onychauxis, 58t
Onychogryphosis, 58t, 225
Onycholysis, 58t
Onychomycosis, 58t
Opening snaps, 151, 152
Ophthalmic nerve (CN V1), *91*, 92
Oppenheim's reflex, 249t
Optic nerve (CN II), 81t, 83–84
Oral cavity, 77–80
Orchitis, 270
Orientation, 228, 232
Oropharynx, 80
Orthostatic hypotension, 43–44, 44t
Orthostatic pulse measurement, 41–45
Orthostatic tachycardia, 43
Osler nodes, 194
Osteoarthrosis, 101, 263
Osteomalacia, 264
Osteoporosis, 263
Otitis externa, 75
Otitis media, 75
Ovaries
    enlargement of, 289
    palpation of, 284
    size of, 289

Paget's disease
    of bone, 67, 202
    of breast, 63t, 121

Pain
    abdominal, 173, 177–184
    facial, 90
    lower back, 255–262
    superficial perception of, 236
Palate, 78
Palpation, 10
Pancreas, 169
Pancreatitis, 183t–184t, 184
Papanicolaou smear, 118, 277, 291, *292*
Papilledema, 233
Papules, 51, 56t
    penile, 267
Paranasal sinuses, 76–77
    percussion of, 77
    transillumination of, 77, *78*
Paraphimosis, 268
Paraspinal muscles, 251, 254
Parkinsonism, 208, 244
Paronychia, 58t
Parotid enlargement, 68
Passive straight-leg raising maneuver, 159
Past medical history (PMH), 4–6
Past-pointing, 250
Patch, 50
Patellar reflex, 246, 261
Patient profile (PP), 6–7
Patrick's test, 263
Pectoriloquy, 139
Pectus carinatum, 126
Pectus excavatum, 126
Pemphigoid, bullous, 57t
Pemphigus vulgaris, 57t
Penis, 265–268
    poor hygiene, 266–267
    skin conditions of, 267
    squamous cell carcinoma of, 267
    swelling of, 268

Penis–*continued*
  trauma of, 267
Percussion, 10
Perianal skin problems, 64t,
    273–274, 288
Pericardial rubs, 150, 157
Periodontitis, 79
Periorbital structures. *See* Eye
    and periorbital structures
Peripheral nerves, *240–241*
Peripheral neuropathy, 235, 239t
Peristalsis, 182
Peritonitis, 182, 183t–184t
Peroneal nerves, 225
Pes cavus, 223
Pes equinus, 223
Pes planus, 223
Petechiae, 50
Peyronie's disease, 268
Pfannenstiel incision, *171*
Phelan's sign, 209
Phimosis, 268
Physical examination, 9–13
    instruments and supplies for,
        13, 13t
    modes for, 10
    sequence of, 10t–12t
Pigmentation, 54–55
    of areola, 120
    postinflammatory
        hyperpigmentation, 65t
Pigmented bands, 58t
Pilocarpine, 86
Plantar flexion, 221
Plantar response, 248–249, 249t
Plaques
    skin, 51, 56t
    on tongue, 79
Pleural rubs, 136
Point of maximal impulse, 142
Pollution, 25

Polymastia, 120
Polythelia, 120
Popliteal fossa, 213
Posterior cruciate ligament,
    219–220
Pregnancy
    breasts during, 120–122
    location of cardiac impulse
        during, 142–143
    pelvic examination in,
        292
    ruptured ectopic, 184t
Pregnancy and delivery history,
    6
Premature atrial contractions,
    146
Premature ejaculation, 17
Premature ventricular
    contractions, 146
Prognathia, 68
Proprioceptive dysfunction,
    244
Prostate, *266*, 275–276
Prostate cancer, 276
Prostatitis, 276
Proverb interpretation, 228
Pseudomonas infection, 60t, 65t
Psoriasis, 56t, 267
Ptosis, 69
Pubic crest, 169
Pulmonic insufficiency, 155,
    161
Pulmonic stenosis, 143, 150
Pulse, 34t–35t, 35–36
    brachial, 194
    carotid, 142, 162–164,
        166–167
    dorsalis pedis, 210
    femoral, 192
    orthostatic, 41–45
    popliteal, 210, *211*
    posterior tibial, 210

radial, 35t, 195t
ulnar, 195
Pulse pressure, 35
Pulsus paradoxus, 35–36,
    45–46, 46t
Pupils
    accommodation, 85–86
    anisocoria, 69, 87
    Argyll Robertson, 87
    dilation of, 72–73
    drugs affecting size of, 86
    light reflex, 85, *85*, 86
    Marcus Gunn, 88
Purpura, 50
    cardiologist's, 194
    fulminans, 60t
    pinch, 194
Push-off test, 208–209
Pustule, 52
Pyelonephritis, 129
Pyorrhea, 79

Quadrant test, 103
Queen Anne's sign, 59t, 68

Rales, 136
Ram's horn nails, 225
Rape examination, 293
Raynaud's phenomenon, 196
Reasoning, 228
Rebound tenderness, 179
Recreational drug use history, 6
    extended, 21–22
Rectal examination. *See*
    Anorectal examination
Rectal prolapse, 273, 275
Rectovaginal septum, 291
Rectus abdominis muscle, 173
Reflex sympathetic dystrophy,
    212
Reflex(es), 245–247, *246–247*,
    248t

abdominal, 248–249
Achilles, 246–247, *247*
Babinski's, 249
biceps, 246
brachioradialis, 246
Chaddock, 249t
cremasteric, 249
Gordon, 249t
levels of, 248t
muscle stretch, 235, 245–247,
    246–247, 248t
Oppenheim's, 249t
patellar, 246
plantar, 248
pupillary light, 85, *85*, 86
Schäfer's, 249t
superficial, 248–249, 249t
triceps, 245–246
Reiter's syndrome, 267
Renal artery stenosis, 192
Respiration, 125–128. *See also*
    Lung
    abnormal breath sounds,
        135–136
    cycled respiration test, 160
    forced expiratory time, 138
    normal breath sounds, 135t
    rate of, 36, 126
    rhythm of, 126
Respiratory distress, 36t
Retina, 72
Retinal venous pulsations, 233
Retroperitoneal irritation, 184
Review of systems (ROS), 7–9
Rheumatoid arthritis, 207
Rheumatoid nodules, 203, 204
Rhinitis, 76–77
Ribs
    springing test of, 128, 129
    tenderness of, 129
Riedel's thyroiditis, 106
Rinne test, 93, 95, 96t

Rocky Mountain spotted fever, 60t
Romberg test, 208, 237–239
Rosacea, 62t

S_1, 146–148, *147*
  absence of, 146
  "double," 146
  split, 146–147
  unduly loud, 147–148
  variable intensity of, 146
S_2, *147*, 148–149
  audible expiratory splitting
    of, 149
  fixed splitting of, 149
  loud, 148
  loud S_2P, 148
  normal physiologic splitting
    of, 148
  paradoxical splitting of, 149
  soft, 148
S_3, *151*, 151–152
S_4, 146–147, *151*, 151–152
Sacroiliac joint, 254
Sarcoidosis, 110, 204
Scales, 51, 56t
Scapular winging, 209
Schäfer's reflex, 249t
Schober's flexion test, 256, *259*
Sciatic nerve lesion, 225, 261
Sciatic notch palpation, 258
Scoliosis, 127, 251, 252
Screening examination, 1–13
  medical history, 1–9
  physical examination, 9–13
Scrotum, 265–268
  empty, 269
  masses and transillumination
    of, 270–272, *271*
  palpation of, 268–270
  swelling of, 268

Sensory evaluation, 230–231, 236–239
  bilateral simultaneous
    stimulation, 237
  interpretation of, 237–239
  joint position sense, 236
  light touch, 236
  Romberg test, 237
  sensory deficits, 236–237, 239t
  superficial pain, 236
  temperature perception, 237
  vibratory sense, 236
Septic arthritis, 224
Seventh nerve palsy, 92–93
Sexual history, 7
  extended, 15–20
    attitude for, 16
    concerns common to men
      and women, 18
    concerns raised by physical
      examination, 19–20
    concerns specific to men,
      17–18
    concerns specific to
      women, 18–19
    indications for, 15–16
    sexual issues raised by
      history of present
      illness, 16–17
Sexual responsiveness, lack of, 18
Sexually transmitted diseases, 267, 274
Shingles, 57t
Shoes, 224
Shoulder, 197–202
  Apley scratch test of, 201t
  loss of convexity of, 202
  muscle and nerve control of
    motion of, 201t
  reduced power in, 200–201

testing range of motion of, 197, *198–200*
unilateral dropped, 201
Sickle cell anemia, 67
Sign
    anterior drawer, 220
    black bottom, 274
    blue genital sign of Bryant, 268
    Brudzinski's contralateral reflex, 234t
    Brudzinski's nape of neck, 234t
    Carvallo's, 160
    Chadwick's, 291
    Cullen's, 184
    Dahl's, 125
    Dickinson's, 291
    digiti quinti, 239, 243
    frontal lobe, 231t
    Gottron's, 206
    Grey Turner's, 184
    heliotrope, 62t
    Kernig's, 234t
    knuckle, 207
    Kussmaul's, 168
    ladder, 182
    Lasègue, 234t
    Murphy's, 180, 184
    "neck," 101
    Phelan's, 209
    posterior drawer, 220
    Queen Anne's, 59t, 68
    Tinel's, 209
Sinus arrhythmia, 146
Sinus bradycardia, 35t, 145
Sinus rhythm, 145
Sinus tachycardia, 145–146
Sinusitis, 77
Skene's glands, 280
Skin examination, 47–65
    interpretation of, 48–55

abnormalities localized to back, perineum, perianal, and genital areas, 64t
abnormalities localized to breasts and axillae, 63t
abnormalities localized to head and neck, 62t
abnormalities localized to legs and feet, 65t
alterations in skin texture, 55
body location and distribution, 53, *53–54*
characteristics of lesions, *48–49*
depressed lesions, *52–53*, 56t
diascopy, 54
flat lesions, *49–50*, 55t
hair alterations, 59t
hemorrhagic rashes and lesions in febrile patients, 60t
malignant melanoma, 63t
nail alterations, 58t
pressure ulcers, 64t
raised cystic lesions, *52*, 57t
raised solid lesions, *51–52*, 56t
skin color, 54–55
widespread abnormalities, 61t
Wood's light findings, 54, 65t
techniques for, 47–48
    diascopy, 48
    inspection, 47
    magnification, 48
    palpation, 47
    Wood's light, 48

Skin tags, 56t, 63t, 290
Small bowel obstruction, 179, 182, 183t
Snellen eye chart, 83
Solar elastosis, 62t
Spasticity, 242
Speculum examination, 280–284, *281, 283*
Speech, 228–231
Spider angioma, 50
Spinal cord, 234–235, *235,* 239t
Spinal curvatures, 252–254, *253*
Spinal fractures, 264
Spinal nerve roots, 234–235, *235,* 239t
 cervical root disease, 103–104
 lower back pain and dysfunction of, 258–261, 260t
Spinal osteoarthrosis, 263
Spinal range of motion, 254, *255–256*
Spinal stenosis, 261, 264
Spleen, 170, 177
Splenomegaly, 174, 188
Spondyloarthropathy, 256
Spondylolisthesis, 263
Spots
 café-au-lait, 55t
 "cotton-wool," 72
 Fordyce, 64t, 268
 Roth, 72
 shin, 65t
Spousal abuse, 22
Staphylococcal bacteremia, 60t
Steppage gait, 225
Stereognosis, 231
Stethoscope, 143
Stocking pattern, 235
Stomach, 169
Stomatitis, 79
Stoop test, 261

Straight-leg raising, 259
 crossed, 259
 passive, 159
 reverse, 261
"Stretch marks," 55t
Striae, 55t
Stupor, 233
Subclavian artery stenosis, 194
Subclavian steal syndrome, 194–195
Substance use history, 6
 extended, 20–22
Suicidal thoughts, 24
Sun exposure, 55
Supraclavicular fossa, 108–109, *109*
Surgical procedures, 4
Symptoms, 3–4
Syphilis, 110, 267
Systemic lupus erythematosus, 60t, 196, 204
Systemic sclerosis, 197
Systole, 150

Tachycardia
 fever without, 38t
 orthostatic, 43
 sinus, 145–146
Tachypnea, 126
Tactile perception, 230–231, 236
Tactile vocal fremitus, 136–138, *137*
Tanner stages of breast development, *116*
Tardive dyskinesia, 242
Teeth, 78
Telangiectases, 55t
 palatal, 80
Temperature measurement, 36–37
Temperature perception, 237

Testes, 268
  abnormalities of, 269
  atrophy of, 269
  cancer of, 271
  masses of, 270–272, *271*
  palpation of, 269
  size of, 269
  undescended, 269
Thermometers, 36–37
Thomas' test, 217–219
Thorax, 125–139. *See also* Lung
  auscultation of lung, 134–136
  chest wall observation, 125–128
  forced expiratory time, 138
  palpation for tactile vocal fremitus, 136–138, *137*
  palpation of bony thorax, 128–129
    at costovertebral angle, 129
    for subcutaneous emphysema, 129
    technique for, 128–129
  percussion of lung, 130–134
  surface projections
    of bony structures, *126*
    of posterior viscera, *128*
    of right pulmonary lobes, *127*
Thrills, 142, 143
Thumb motion, 202t
Thyroid gland, *99, 105,* 105–106
Ticklishness, 173
Tics, 243
Timolol, 86
Tinea pedis, 65t
Tinea versicolor, 65t
Tinel's sign, 209
Tinetti functional test, 215, 216t, 244

Tobacco use, 6
Toes, 223–225
  deformities of, 224
  maceration between, 224
  muscle and nerve control of motion of, 217t
  other tests of, 223–225
  plantar flexion of, 221
  toenail disorders, 223–225
Tongue, 77–79
  deviation of, 97–98
  glossitis, 79
  hemiatrophy or fasciculation of, 98
Torsion of appendix testis, 270
Torticollis, 100
Toxin exposure, 26
Toxoplasmosis, 110
Trachea, *99,* 112, 125
Tracheal tug, 112
Transient arterial occlusion maneuver, 160–161
Transillumination
  of paranasal sinuses, 77, *78*
  of scrotal masses, 270–272, *271*
Trauma, 5
  abuse, 22
  sexual, 20, 292–293
Tremor, 242–243
  hand, 208, 208t
  rest vs. intention, 208
Trendelenburg position, 166
Trendelenburg test, 216–217, *218*
Triceps reflex, 245–246
Tricuspid regurgitation, 167
Tricuspid stenosis, 166
Trigeminal nerve (CN V), 81t, 90–92, *91*
Trochlear nerve (CN IV), 81t, 88–90

Tuberculosis, 110, 134
Tumor. *See also* Cancer,
    carcinoma; Masses
  Pancoast, 134
  skin, 51
Turner's syndrome, 100
Tympanic membrane, *74, 75*
Typhus, 60t

Ulcers
  diabetic foot, 65t, 223, 224
  pressure, 57t, 64t
  skin, 53
  venous, 65t
  vulvar, 287
Ulnar deviation, 205, 206
Upper limb, 194–210
  arterial, venous, and
      capillary circulation of,
      194–197
  joints, tendons, muscles, and
      bones of, 197–207
    elbow, 203–204
    hand and fingers, 205–207
    muscle and nerve control
        of joint motion, 201t–202t
    shoulder, 197–202, *198–200*
    wrist, 204
  lymphatic drainage of, 197
  other tests of, 208–210
  peripheral nerves and
      muscles of, 207, 249–250
  tremor in, 208, 208t
Upper motor neuron lesions,
    243, 243t
Ureteral calculus, 184
Urethral meatus
  female, 287
  male, 265
Urethral rupture, 268
Urethritis, 267

Urinary bladder, 171, 177
  distension of, 189
Uterine cervix, 280–284, *281, 283*
  abnormalities of, 288
  palpation of, 284
Uterus
  abnormalities of, 289
  palpation of, 284, *285*
  positions of, 289, *290*
  prolapse of, 289

Vagina
  abnormalities of, 287, 288
  atrophy of, 20, 288
  inspection of, 280–284, *281,
      283*
Vagus nerve (CN X), 81t, 96–97
Valsalva maneuver, 157–158
Varicella, 57t
Varicocele, 272
Varicose veins, 213
Vas deferens, 269, 270
Vasectomy, 270
Vasitis nodosum, 270
Venous hums, cervical,
    104–105, 164
Venous "spider," 50
Ventricular hypertrophy
  left, 142, 143
  right, 142, 167
Verbal expression, 230
Vertebrobasilar insufficiency,
    194
Vesicle, 52, 57t
Vestibular dysfunction, 93–94
Vibratory sense, 236, 237
Violence in family, 22–23
Visual acuity testing, 83
Visual agnosia, 234
Visual field defects, 84, 234
Visual field testing, 83
Visual perception, 231

Vital signs, 34–46
    blood pressure
        measurement, 37–45
    pulse, 34t–35t, 35–36
        pulsus paradoxus, 35–36,
            45–46
    respirations, 36, 36t
    temperature measurement,
        36–37
Vitamin D deficiency, 126
Vitiligo, 55t, 65t
Volvulus, 182
Vulva, 279–280, *280*, 287
Vulvar dystrophies, 64t
Vulvitis, atrophic, 64t
Vulvovaginitis, 20

Warts, 56t
    genital, 64t, 267
Weber test, 93, 95, 96t
Weight changes, 26–27
Wernicke's aphasia, 230
Wheal, 51
Wheezing, 112, 136
Wood's light examination, 48,
    54, 65t
Work exposures, 25
Wrist, 202t, 204
Written expression, 230
Wryneck, 100

Xanthomas, 56t, 204